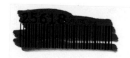

OXFORD

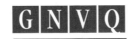

Intermediate
HEALTH & SOCIAL CARE

This book is to be returned on or before
the last date st

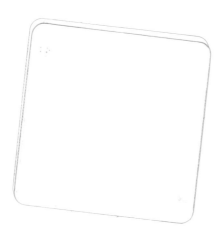

Christine Barratt

OXFORD
UNIVERSITY PRESS

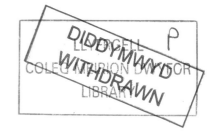

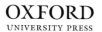

OXFORD
UNIVERSITY PRESS

Oxford University Press, Great Clarendon Street, Oxford OX2 6DP

Oxford   New York

Athens Auckland Bangkok Bogota Buenos Aires
Calcutta Cape Town Chennai Dar es Salaam
Delhi Florence Hong Kong Istanbul Karachi
Kuala Lumpur Madras Madrid Melbourne
Mexico City Mumbai Nairobi Paris São Paulo
Shanghai Singapore Taipei Tokyo Toronto Warsaw

and associated companies in
Berlin Ibadan

Oxford is a trade mark of Oxford University Press

First published 1996 Reprinted 1998
Second edition 2000

ISBN 0 19 832830 3

Typesetting and page layout by Ruth Nason and Carole Binding

Illustration by Hilary Earl, David Huggins, Gordon Lawson, Peter Marsh,
Oxford Illustrators, Geo Parkin, Julie Tolliday and Lynn Williams.

Printed in Spain by Gráficas Estella, S. A.

*The publisher would like to thank the following for their kind permission to
reproduce the following photographs:*

Ace Photo Agency **page 157 bl** Michael Bluestone; Anthony Blake Photo
Library/Andrew Sydenham **page 97 c**; A-Z Botanical **page 70 l** Jiri Loun,
page 70 cl W. Broadhurst, **page 70 cr** Steven Owens, **page 70 r** F. Merlet;
Collections **page 137 al & ar** Anthea Sieveking; Food Features **page 97 l**,
97 r; Format **page 25** Miriam Reik, **page 39 a** Maggie Murray, **page 93**
Maggie Murray, **page 136** Joanne O'Brien, **page 137 bl** Jacky Chapman,
page 156 Judy Harrison; Sally Greenhill **page 39 b, 112, 116 al, 137 br**;
Richard Greenhill **page 57**; Health Education Authority **page 116 bl**;
Photofusion **page 63** Liam Bailey, **page 146** Robert Brook; Courtesy
Rexam Medical Packaging **page 102**; RNIB **page 24 l** Tony Sleep,
page 24 r Sally Lancaster, **page 39 c** Sally Lancaster; TRIP **page 157 al**
J. Highet, **page 157 ar** J. Wakelin, **page 157 br** P. Rauter.

Key **a** - above; **b** - below; **l** - left; **r** - right; **c** - centre.

Cover photo - Collections/Anthea Sieveking

*The publisher would like to thank the staff and students of Abingdon College
for trialling some of the text.*

Contents

Dedication

I would like to dedicate this book to Sarah, our daughter.

Introduction

About the GNVQ

The General National Vocational Qualification in Health and Social Care offers you a wide background knowledge of work in this occupational field. Gaining a certificate for the Intermediate level will equip you to

1 apply for a job

2 progress to further study, such as Advanced level GNVQ or GCSE A level subjects, and then into higher education at college or university

3 work towards a National Vocational Qualification (NVQ). The two especially relevant NVQs are in Care, and Early Years Care and Education.

To gain an Intermediate GNVQ in Health and Social Care, you will have to complete the three mandatory units covered in this book. There are also units called optional units; they are not covered in this book because they vary according to which of the three awarding bodies – AQA, Edexcel Foundation, or OCR – designs them. You will select from the optional units of the awarding body with which you are registered by your school or college. Your teacher or lecturer will explain the choices to you and guide you through them.

A full Intermediate level GNVQ cannot be gained without completing all three mandatory units. But you can get a separate certificate for each individual unit achieved.

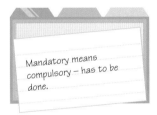

Mandatory means compulsory – has to be done.

Assessment

Assessment involves judgement and grading. The three mandatory units are judged and graded by

- **internal** assessment by your school or college
- **external** assessment by your awarding body.

For the internal assessment (two-thirds of the total possible marks) you have to collect a **portfolio** of evidence of your ability and knowledge for Units 1 and 2. Your portfolio will be internally assessed in your school or college, and the assessment will be confirmed by a representative of the awarding body, who is called an external verifier.

The other third of the total possible marks come from external assessment of work relating to Unit 3 that the awarding body sets and marks. But you will still need to collect evidence of your learning in your portfolio, as a back-up for this external assessment.

It is possible to gain a **pass**, **merit**, or **distinction**. You cannot achieve a pass until you have completed your portfolio and been successful in the external assessment. This book aims to provide you with enough knowledge and portfolio evidence to enable you to achieve at least a pass grade, with some extra ideas for how to gain higher grades. Teaching staff will explain to you in more detail how merits and distinctions can be achieved.

Key Skills

As well as your understanding of health and social care, your work can also show your knowledge and use of additional general skills. These are known as **Key Skills**, and are

- communication

- application of number

- information technology.

You can get a Key Skills certificate by completing units on these skills. As you work through this book, you will be examining aspects of the use of these skills in health and social care; and some of the activities suggested offer simple opportunities for you to demonstrate your competence at a basic standard. These activities are indicated with a signpost symbol.

A brief outline of the Key Skills units at level 2 is given in the Key Skills Preface on page 12. The Key Skills are designed on five **levels** – this book concentrates on level 2. If you are particularly advanced in one or all of the Key Skills, it is possible for you to achieve a higher level while completing your Intermediate programme. For this you will need guidance from your teaching staff.

C2.1a, 3.3

The signpost symbol is used throughout the book to indicate activities that will allow you to produce evidence for Key Skills units.

About this book

This book aims to lead you through the knowledge requirements laid down in the three mandatory units, at the same time helping you to put together evidence for your portfolio through activities, case studies, and questions.

The book is in three chapters and each chapter covers one unit. Each chapter has an introduction to the unit content, followed by a pattern of

- knowledge and activities

- case studies

- multiple choice questions *(Note that these are not part of the unit's formal assessment, but are included so that you can test your knowledge for yourself.)*

- compulsory assessment activities

- summary of evidence opportunities
- personal evidence tracking record.

Knowledge and activities

For each unit, activities are suggested which will enable you to gather evidence of your knowledge and understanding. Each piece of evidence will need to be placed in your portfolio with a reference number. The personal tracking record will help with this.

Ideas are included for presenting the suggested evidence, using Key Skills techniques, but you will need specialist help from your teacher or lecturer for completing the Key Skills' own units. Aspects of all three skills – communication, application of number, and information technology – that are important for you to understand before you begin are outlined in the Key Skills Preface (page 12).

The symbol ◆ indicates **extension opportunities**. These give you the chance to extend your understanding and knowledge of a particular area. Take advantage of them if you are aiming for a merit or distinction grade; it will show that you are prepared to work independently. They will also give you ideas for developing other activities further if you wish to. Remember that the signpost symbol is used to indicate **Key Skills opportunities**.

Case studies

The case studies are based on four fictitious organisations:

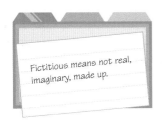

Fictitious means not real, imaginary, made up.

1 Netherfield Community Care team

2 Hill Hall, a school for children and young adults with profound learning difficulties

3 The Thatched Cottage residential care home

4 Down Way School.

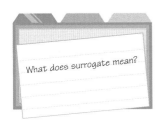

What does surrogate mean?

These four establishments, described in detail on page 8, will provide you with surrogate placements if you are not able to visit care organisations on your course of study. The scenarios described are intended to be as realistic as possible, all examples being drawn from actual care work experiences.

Summary of evidence opportunities and personal evidence tracking record

The evidence opportunities provided for each unit are summarised in a table at the end of the unit chapter (for example, page 84). These 'summary of evidence' tables enable you to see at a glance where the text has given you the opportunity to produce evidence. On a photocopy of the personal tracking record you will be able to fill in a description of your evidence as it is produced, and see where you need to do further work. There is space too for the reference number of your evidence, to help you with the organisation of your portfolio.

The GNVQ system encourages students **to take responsibility for their own learning**. The activities suggested in the book offer you the opportunity to produce evidence of your understanding of the Health and Social Care units as already described. You may choose to expand on these activities. Remember that books like this one are not your only resources. Television, newspapers, radio, films, and magazines constantly discuss the matters of human interest on which your GNVQ units focus.

Look at your own and your friends' and family's life experiences. Bring these to bear in your evidence, which will become more lively and realistic, up-to-date, and thoughtful. You must, of course, make sure that any facts you choose to present are from an accurate and reliable source, and that, if the people involved are friends or clients, you get their permission to use their experiences in this way.

Confidentiality is a key issue in the field of health and social care. It is covered specifically in Unit 1, but is worth a mention here in the context of case studies and work experience. Every student must be aware of the need for confidentiality in all aspects of caring, including any written work which may follow visits outside the school or college. This will have to be discussed with your teacher or lecturer, and the supervisor in any place of work.

You will find **'fact file-cards'** scattered throughout the book. These are intended to clarify words and phrases used in the text. You might like to keep a glossary or dictionary of the most useful; many will help to expand your professional language.

The case study establishments

Netherfield Community Care

Netherfield is a sprawling urban area. It has expanded from an industrial heartland to encompass several surrounding villages. The community is mixed, ranging from an ageing local population through a strong Polish community to young people attracted to small, affordable high-rise flats. Some areas of the town are depressed.

A community team works in this environment. The Community Care Act has increased the team's responsibilities considerably. There have always been clients who very much preferred to stay independent in their own homes despite requiring care, but now several hostels for people with mental health problems have opened. The Netherfield community team is responding by taking on trained staff able to meet this new need.

Mikhail

Debbie

8

The members of the community care team feel that community care work is very rewarding, demanding, and stimulating, and are keen to encourage people to consider it as a career. With this in mind they welcome students from Netherfield College on work placement, both those straight from school and mature students.

The health care worker who organises the work experience of students is Mikhail, a young Polish national. He is an idealist, but his training has made his attitude more realistic without quashing his dreams.

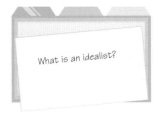

What is an idealist?

He transmits his enthusiasm for community care to the students he supervises. He is dedicated to improving the quality of life for all clients while naturally relating well to the Polish community. His English is almost perfect.

Debbie is a student who loves the variety given by community care. She is distressed by the financial restraints affecting services, and is resisting Mikhail's attempts to encourage her to accept the situation without causing a fuss.

Hill Hall

Hill Hall is a school catering for children from 3 to 19 years of age from a wide surrounding area, who arrive by bus, taxi, and private transport each day. All the children have severe learning difficulties, and require constant care alongside their education. The school aims to provide the opportunity for all pupils to meet their potential. Most will never be able to integrate into society. Some die while they are still children. Others succeed against all odds. Staff are somewhat dissatisfied. The school is very expensive to maintain and it is rumoured that it will close in five years' time.

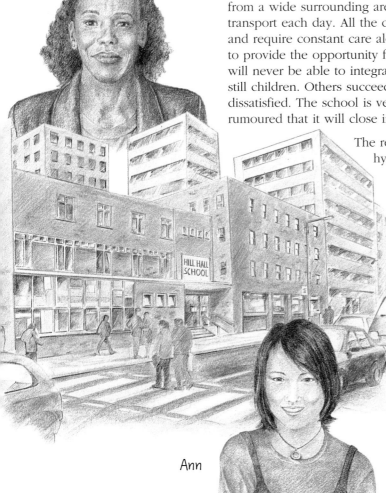

Molly

Ann

The resources are excellent – including a hydrotherapy bath and a Schnoozlen room in which children can listen to gentle music and experience a variety of lighting effects and different touch and smell sensations in complete safety. The dedicated staff are skilled in meeting all the pupils' needs, including physiotherapy and special diets.

The school is set in the centre of a city and welcomes students from the local college for work experience, although it is aware that the work makes special demands. The severity of the children's disabilities can be difficult for some carers to come to terms with.

Molly is a dedicated senior care worker, who has worked in the school team for

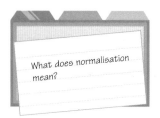

What does normalisation mean?

many years. She is devoted to the children, and is committed to the normalisation process. She is the person to whom placement students naturally turn, as she is approachable and sympathetic.

The student at present on placement at Hill Hall is Ann, who is very new to this type of work and finding it hard to come to grips with the severity of the children's disabilities. She is quiet and does not share her anxieties easily. Her first inclination is to go off sick when things alarm her, but she is trying to overcome this. She sleeps badly, as she worries about her attitude and wonders if she has chosen the wrong course.

The Thatched Cottage

The Thatched Cottage is a residential home by the sea. It has 23 residents, mostly elderly. Some have been transferred from a local hospital for people with moderate learning disabilities, which has recently closed down.

Some residents are able-bodied, while others are handicapped by a variety of complaints ranging from arthritis to chronic bronchitis. Some are confused, others are alert. Public transport is limited. There is a pub, a post office, and a few shops nearby, with a tea-room up the road. The nearest churches are about a mile away. The ground falls steeply to the sea outside the house. The gardens are big enough to hold summer fetes and other activities, but not flat enough for residents with mobility problems to stroll far.

Dora

In addition to its usual staff, The Thatched Cottage welcomes college and secondary school pupils on work experience, and has other staff on employment training.

Dora is the senior care assistant in The Thatched Cottage. She has ten years' experience, and has recently been put in charge of managing new care assistants and all those working on a temporary or short-term basis in the home. She is therefore the line manager of students on placement.

You will be following the progress of Mark, a student from the local college. He is not sure what he wants to do after completing his course, but enjoys working with the residents as it gives him a wide range of caring experience. He knows that it will come in useful, and will also strengthen his letters of application for work.

Mark

A line manager is someone responsible for certain other workers, from whom they can seek guidance and advice.

Down Way School

Isabel

Jalwinder

Down Way School is a rural primary school. It was built in Edwardian times and many of the children's parents attended in their childhood. The number of pupils has fallen recently. Now that there is room for it, the school has opened a small nursery/playgroup in one of its biggest classrooms. A new housing estate is being developed nearby, and the children living there will attend Down Way next September.

There are at present 106 children, the youngest being two and a half and the oldest eleven. When they leave, the older children move on to the local comprehensive school about a mile away. Young people who used to attend the school return to Down Way for work experience, and college students also visit on a placement basis for vocational courses.

Isabel is a non-teaching assistant at the school. She began helping voluntarily as a mother when her children were small, and later gained a part-time post; she now works full time. She knows a great deal about the school, and has moved about into different classes as the school has changed. She is very much looking forward to seeing numbers grow, and has helped a great deal with the development of the nursery, as she has had playgroup experience.

Jalwinder is a Punjabi health care student on placement at Down Way. She wants to run her own nursery school eventually. She is a cheerful, competent girl and finds her creative skills useful when working with the children.

Now read on. Enjoy your studies. In the end they will enable you to enter into a lifetime of stimulating and rewarding work in one of the caring professions.

Key Skills Preface

1 Communication

This unit is about applying your communication skills to deal with straightforward subjects and extended written material.

You must	Evidence must show that you can
C2.1a – contribute to a discussion about a straightforward subject	• make clear and relevant contributions in a way that suits your purpose and situation • listen and respond appropriately to what others say • help to move the discussion forward
C2.1b – give a short talk about a straightforward subject, using an image	• speak clearly in a way that suits your subject, purpose, and situation • keep to the subject and structure your talk to help listeners follow what you are saying • use an image to clearly illustrate your main points
C2.2 – read and summarise information from **two** extended documents about a straightforward subject (One of the documents should include at least **one** image.)	• select and read relevant materials • identify accurately the lines of reasoning and main points from text and images • summarise the information to suit your purpose

You must	Evidence must show that you can
C2.3 – write **two** different types of documents about straightforward subjects (One piece of writing should be an extended document and include at least **one** image.)	• present relevant information in an appropriate form • use a structure and a style of writing to suit your purpose • ensure text is legible and that spelling, punctuation, and grammar are accurate, so that your meaning is clear

2 Application of Number

This unit is about applying your number skills in a substantial activity that involves a series of straightforward tasks.

You must	Evidence must show that you can
N2.1 – interpret information from **two** different sources, including material containing a graph	• choose how to obtain the information needed to meet the purpose of the activity • obtain the relevant information • select appropriate methods to get the results you need
N2.2 – carry out calculations to do with: a. amounts and sizes b. scales and proportion c. handling statistics d. using formulae	• carry out calculations, clearly showing your methods and levels of accuracy • check your methods to identify and correct any errors, and make sure your results make sense
N2.3 – interpret the results of your calculations and present your findings (You must use at least **one** graph, **one** chart, and **one** diagram.)	• select effective ways to present your findings • present your findings clearly and describe your methods • explain how the results of your calculations meet the purpose of your activity

3   Information Technology

This unit is about applying your IT skills to suit different purposes.

You must	Evidence must show that you can
IT2.1 – search for and select information for **two** different purposes	<ul><li>identify the information you need and suitable sources</li><li>carry out effective searches</li><li>select information that is relevant to your purpose</li></ul>
IT2.2 – explore and develop information, and derive new information, for **two** different purposes	<ul><li>enter and bring together information using formats that help development</li></ul>
IT2.3 – present combined information for **two** different purposes. (Your work must include at least **one** example of text, **one** example of images, and **one** example of numbers.)	<ul><li>select and use appropriate layouts for presenting combined information in a consistent way</li><li>develop the presentation to suit your purpose and the types of information</li><li>ensure your work is accurate, clear, and saved appropriately</li></ul>

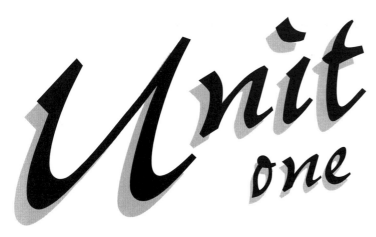

Health, Social Care, and Early Years Provision

Introduction

In this unit you will learn about

- the main roles of people who work in the health, social care, and early years services, and the structures within which they function
- the care value base that underpins all health and social care work with clients
- the skills that are needed by people working in the health, social care, and early years services
- the basic communication skills that are needed by people working in the health, social care, and early years services.

This unit is assessed through your portfolio work, and the grade you are given will be your grade for the unit.

What you need to know		
1	The organisation of health, social care, and early years services	16
2	The main jobs in health, social care, and early years services	23
3	Effective communication skills	37
4	The care value base	55
5	Codes of practice and charters	81

Unit 1.1
The organisation of health, social care, and early years services

To help you to understand how services are organised into different categories or sectors, you will need to identify examples of services, in different sectors, in your own locality. The different sectors are

- statutory
- voluntary
- private
- informal.

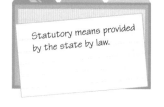

Statutory means provided by the state by law.

Summary of provision of health and social care

Category or sector	Explanation	Examples
Statutory	Provided by the state; that is, services which must be provided by law	NHS Local authority services
Voluntary	Privately organised, often non-profit-making. Filling gaps in state provision	NSPCC, Mind, Help the Aged, Terence Higgins Trust
Private	Privately owned and run on business lines – profit-making	Private hospitals, private residential care, nursing homes, childminders
Informal	Provided by the family and community, friends, neighbours, local support groups	Family care of disabled child Day services provided by a church group

The statutory sector

The National Health Service (NHS) and local authority social services together form the two branches of the **statutory** services. Both are controlled nationally by the Secretary of State for Health.

The National Health Service
The care given by the NHS may be primary care, secondary care, or tertiary care.

The people whom you meet first when you need looking after by the National Health Service offer you **primary care**. Often this is in your GP's surgery or at a health clinic, and the people involved include the GP, the practice nurse, and the health visitor.

Sometimes primary care is **preventive**, which may mean that advice is given to stop someone becoming unwell. Two examples are the promotion of how to stop smoking and pre-natal care to make sure that a pregnant woman remains in the best possible health until her baby is born. Primary care is always given outside hospitals, in the community.

Secondary care is always given in hospitals. If you went to an Accident and Emergency department of a hospital, you would be going straight into secondary care. If your GP referred you to a hospital consultant, you would be moving from primary into secondary care. Secondary care is usually **curative**, which means it is intended to make you better, or improve your state of health.

The stage following secondary care is called **tertiary care**, tertiary meaning third. It refers to long-term care, which includes rehabilitation.

Rehabilitation is care intended to restore people to health, or to help them to live as fully as possible within the limits of their personal state of health. This includes, for example,

- those who have had a stroke who may be in tertiary care while they adjust to reduced mobility
- people who have suffered spinal injury who might remain in tertiary care until their condition is stable and they have learnt how to manage ordinary household tasks from a wheelchair.

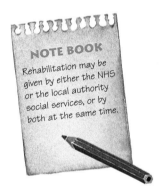

NOTE BOOK

Rehabilitation may be given by either the NHS or the local authority social services, or by both at the same time.

Local authority social services

The role of social services is to give advice, give access to services, and provide some services, including community and residential care. Local authority social services departments purchase services from the full range of statutory and non-statutory providers.

Personal social services make provision for

- families
- children
- young people
- adults
- clients with physical disabilities
- people with learning difficulties and disabilities
- elderly people.

The organisers responsible for delivering care have to work together to make sure that standards are high and that money is spent wisely.

A 'young person' is defined by social services as an individual between the ages of 16 and 18.

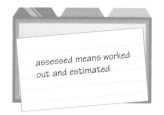

assessed means worked out and estimated

In order to make sure that providers are chosen effectively, the needs of clients have to be **assessed** carefully.

Community services are provided by local authority social services or by the NHS, or by both working together. Their aim is to deliver care within the community or in the clients' own homes. Workers in the area of community service include

- community nurses
- social services field workers
- community psychiatric nurses
- midwives.

ACTIVITY A

Write down the main purpose of each of the four voluntary organisations mentioned in the paragraph on 'The voluntary sector'.

ACTIVITY B

1 Make two lists of care service providers in your area, under the headings 'voluntary' and 'private'.

2 Which list is the longer?

3 Can you draw any conclusions from this?

4 Conduct a survey among a wide cross-section of individuals to ascertain what they consider to be the most important service offered in the two categories.

5 How does the result of your survey compare with local provision as listed in task 1?

6 Discuss the comparison in your group.

C2.1a

The voluntary and private sectors

Services offered by all the different agencies from the **voluntary** and **private** sectors are described as **non-statutory** services. This means that they are not provided by the state.

The voluntary sector

This sector is made up of organisations usually described as charities. They often fill some gap in care which is not totally covered by the statutory services, and include organisations such as Help the Aged and the National Society for the Prevention of Cruelty to Children (NSPCC). Others provide funding, support, or care connected with specific conditions, such as the Terence Higgins Trust and Scope.

The private sector

This sector is made up of organisations run for a profit, such as private hospitals (for example, those run by BUPA), private residential care homes and nursing homes, and private nursery schools, playgroups, and childminding services.

Informal carers

An **informal carer** is one who receives no official payment for services in the form of nursing, companionship, and help in the home. Examples of each of these are

- a husband caring for his wife who suffers from Parkinson's disease
- a neighbour dropping in for coffee and a chat with a housebound friend
- children shopping for invalid parents.

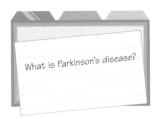

What is Parkinson's disease?

ACTIVITY C

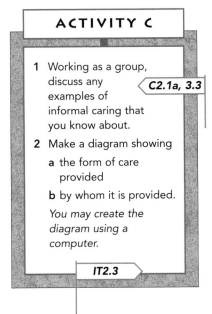

1 Working as a group, discuss any examples of informal caring that you know about. ⟨ *C2.1a, 3.3*

2 Make a diagram showing

   a the form of care provided

   b by whom it is provided.

   You may create the diagram using a computer.

   IT2.3

From these examples it will be easy for you to work out that informal carers include children, parents, friends and neighbours, and local support groups.

Children are a growing group of carers as it becomes more common for people with disabilities to have families. Some children begin in their caring role at a very early age. They may also be expected to help if there is a sibling who needs care in the family. Adult children often look after elderly parents.

Parents are frequently the main carers if a child (or children) needs constant attention.

Friends and neighbours often rally round to help someone who lives alone and is in need of support.

Local support groups can be a source of help to families and individuals, and may be part of a religious or cultural group, or part of a national charity.

Informal carers are entitled to, and are usually deserving of, all the help available from their local community services. This is why you will be examining the types of support available in Unit 3.4 (page 165).

If you choose to go into health and social care work, you may find that members of the public ask you for advice. Again, that same section of Unit 3 will enable you to give information which is accurate and helpful.

ACTIVITY D

◀▶ **Extension opportunity**

1 Find out your local structure of social services.

2 Make a table with actual names of the departments in your area. Compose the diagram using a computer. Save on disk and print.   *IT2.3*

3 You will find long lists of local service providers in the *Yellow Pages*. Make lists under the headings

   • statutory

   • voluntary

   • private

   • support for home carers.

Expand the lists you made in Activity B (page 18).

4 Draw up some relevant questions which would enable you to compare another county's health and social care with your own.
   Conduct a survey based on the criteria you have established.
   When making comparisons you can present graphical illustrations, compare probabilities, and express information in the form of percentages, ratio, and average indicators to support any conclusions made about the two counties.

   N2.3

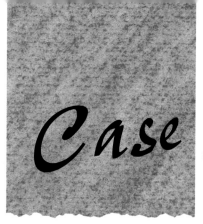

Case Studies

Case study 1.1   Netherfield Community Care

Mikhail is working with the family of Horace, a frail elderly man, to make sure that he remains supported in his wish to stay independent and living alone. He has asked Debbie to make a diagram for him to use when explaining to Horace's relatives the differences between the statutory, voluntary, and private sectors which could contribute to Horace's care.

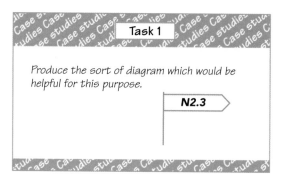

Task 1

Produce the sort of diagram which would be helpful for this purpose.

N2.3

Case study 1.2   Hill Hall

The school is run by the local authority. Ann is surprised at the variety of services used by the pupils and provided by different organisations.

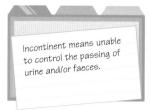

Incontinent means unable to control the passing of urine and/or faeces.

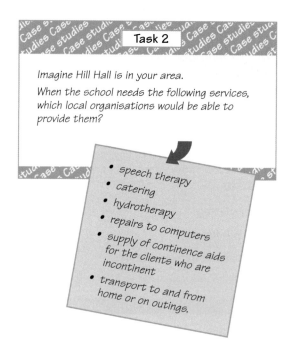

Task 2

Imagine Hill Hall is in your area.

When the school needs the following services, which local organisations would be able to provide them?

- speech therapy
- catering
- hydrotherapy
- repairs to computers
- supply of continence aids for the clients who are incontinent
- transport to and from home or on outings.

Case study 1.3 The Thatched Cottage

Mark comes back from holiday and is surprised to see several clients he doesn't recognise in the sitting room. Dora explains that the management is trying out some new systems in order to help the local community. Midday meals are available to those living nearby, some day-care facilities are being offered, and when accommodation allows, respite care will be offered. Local home carers are enthusiastic.

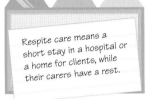

Respite care means a short stay in a hospital or a home for clients, while their carers have a rest.

Task 3

Imagine that The Thatched Cottage is in your area. Make a list of any local organisations offering similar facilities.

Case study 1.4 Down Way School

As part of her course, Jalwinder has to create some printed material which would be of help to new parents. She is keen to make it useful, so she discusses it with Isabel and the class teacher. They suggest that, as there is already a welcome pack for new parents, she should use the opportunity to add to this, outlining the health and social care facilities available for children in the local community.

Task 4

The material should consist of loose leaflets to fit in a folder with a pocket. Working as a group, design the leaflets Jalwinder could produce if she lived in your locality. The leaflets should have words and pictures, all in the same 'house style', covering each of these aspects:

C2.3

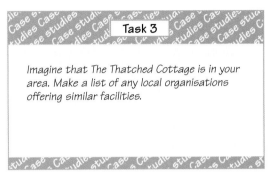

- playgroups
- creches
- health clinics
- holiday child care
- local GPs
- places of worship
- libraries
- mother and toddler groups
- any other matters you consider to be important.

Task 4

Print all the leaflets and save on a disk.

Include a map to show where the main places are, including the Citizens' Advice Bureau, social services, and the nearest post offices.

IT2.3

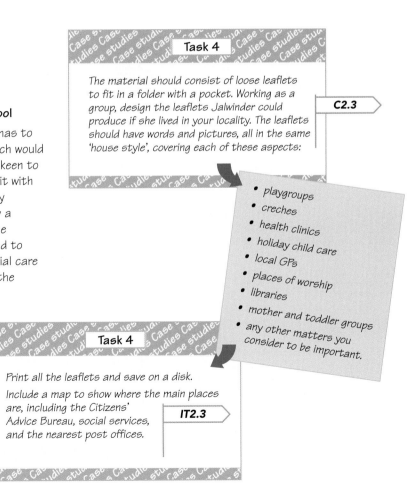

Multiple Choice Questions

1.1 The National Health Services mainly provide

    a *recreational care*

    b *health care*

    c *family care*

    d *community care*

1.2 The services provided by charitable organisations are described as

    a *voluntary*

    b *statutory*

    c *private*

    d *social*

1.3 Which of the following is a provider of care?

    a *local authorities*

    b *the occupational sector*

    c *regional authorities*

    d *the insurance sector*

1.4 Informal carers may meet the needs of clients by

    a *providing statutory care*

    b *forming contracts with local providers*

    c *providing primary health care*

    d *forming local support groups*

Note: These questions are for you to test your knowledge. There is no formal multiple choice test in this GNVQ.

Unit 1.2
The main jobs in health, social care, and early years services

To understand what service workers in health, social care, and early years organisations do, you will need to know their roles. You should understand the roles of staff in different sectors, and the similarities and differences between their work roles. This will include staff who deliver care directly, and those whose work is more indirectly involved with care. Examples are

- **direct care** – nurse, doctor, social worker, care assistant, nursery nurse
- **indirect care** – medical receptionist, cleaner, porter.

Let us first define who needs the help of care service workers.

Clients and client groups, with different needs

The word **client** has developed as a blanket term to describe anybody receiving health and social care. It covers patients in hospital, trainees in sheltered workshops, and all those using health and social care services who have no other neat term to describe them. It is a word with drawbacks, as it is not very warm or friendly, but it is an improvement on 'service user' or 'member of the public'.

When several clients have similar needs and require similar services, they become members of a **client group**: babies, children, young people, adults, elderly people, and families are examples of client groups. The **needs** of these client groups may be

- physical
- emotional
- mental
- social.

For this unit it is not necessary to learn in detail about the needs of different client groups, but the following section will help you to understand better the various demands of care work. You will also find it relevant for Unit 2, when looking at people's needs for positive health.

Physical needs

Clients may have physical needs because of disease, physical disability, or a learning disability.

Disease

Disease can be either **acute** or **chronic**. Acute means short-term, beginning suddenly with a rapid change in the patient's condition, or curable. Chronic means long-term and persistent, with little change from day to day.

Physical disability

Congenital disability   Our bodies are amazingly complex, and it is not surprising that sometimes, during development, things go wrong and babies are born with a disability of one degree or another. Such disabilities are said to be **congenital** and can be for **genetic** reasons (inherited) or **environmental** reasons (damage during development in the womb or at birth).

Acquired disabilities   These are disabilities due to illness or injury after birth.

Congenital and acquired disabilities can be either **motor** – to do with movement, or **sensory** – to do with our senses (sight, hearing, touch, taste, smell).

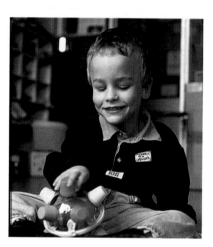

This boy has a congenital disability: he was blind from birth.

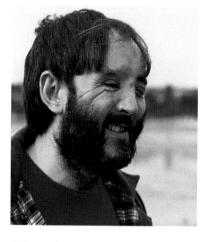

This man has an acquired disability: he lost his sight in an accident.

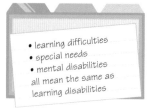

- learning difficulties
- special needs
- mental disabilities

all mean the same as learning disabilities

Learning disability

Usually learning disabilities are recognised in childhood, but sometimes they develop as a result of illness or injuries which affect the brain and stop it functioning normally. Learning disabilities are described as being **moderate** or **severe**, as they range from inability to understand some aspects of daily living to profound dysfunction which could result in death in early adulthood or sooner.

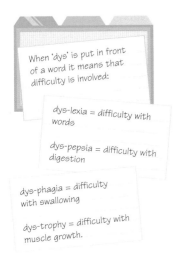

When 'dys' is put in front of a word it means that difficulty is involved:

dys-lexia = difficulty with words

dys-pepsia = difficulty with digestion

dys-phagia = difficulty with swallowing

dys-trophy = difficulty with muscle growth.

Individuals with learning difficulties may or may not have physical disabilities as well. Several terms are used to mean the same as 'learning disability', but it is not now considered acceptable to describe people as 'mentally handicapped'.

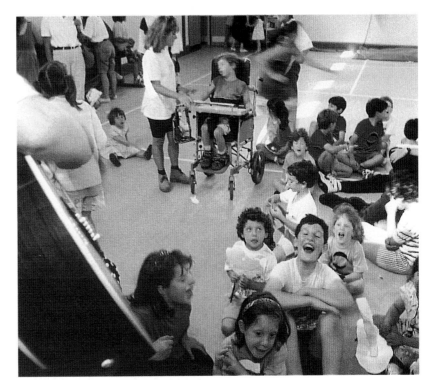

End-of-the-day singing at a centre for children with learning disabilities.

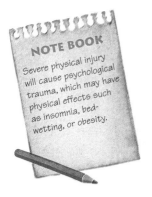

NOTE BOOK

Severe physical injury will cause psychological trauma, which may have physical effects such as insomnia, bed-wetting, or obesity.

Emotional needs

These needs, like physical ones, may be either short-term or long-term, depending on the personality of the client and the nature and extent of the cause. Many emotional needs can be traced back to some past trauma in a client's life. **Trauma** means injury or damage, and it can be either *physical*, as in a cut finger, or *psychological*, as in abuse.

Mental health needs

Mental health is to the mind what physical health is to the body. Just as a physical trauma can be the cause of emotional needs, some physical disorders can show themselves with psychological symptoms. Like physical diseases, mental health disorders can be acute or chronic.

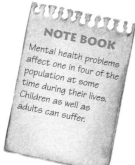

NOTE BOOK

Mental health problems affect one in four of the population at some time during their lives. Children as well as adults can suffer.

Acute For example: behavioural problems caused by food allergies in children; post-natal depression caused by hormone imbalance; aggression caused by uncontrolled diabetes. Mental health needs of this nature are treated through the underlying cause.

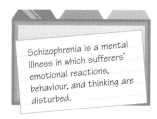

Schizophrenia is a mental illness in which sufferers' emotional reactions, behaviour, and thinking are disturbed.

Chronic   For example, schizophrenia, psychotic behaviour, manic depression, obsessions. Many chronic mental health conditions are manageable with medication, although they may not be curable. It can be a problem to make sure that some sufferers take their prescribed drugs, as sometimes their mental state means that they are not able or inclined to do so.

Social needs

All client groups have social requirements. For example: individuals with physical disabilities may need help with developing self-esteem; families may need support while they adjust to the birth of a baby with disabilities; a child with epilepsy may need guidance through developing friendships. In addition, the main tasks of social service are about supporting families, groups, and all individuals

- financially (with benefits)

- emotionally (with personal contact and advice)

- in material ways (with housing, furniture, etc).

Several client groups will have **educational needs** which will need to be addressed at the same time. Examples are children with special needs, and adults with schizophrenia who choose to go to evening classes.

Carers

Now let us look at those who work with clients and client groups. They are commonly called **carers**, a word covering the numerous jobs in the care field, including health care workers, social workers, volunteers, and those supporting them in various ways.

The everyday work of carers is described, along with the qualifications needed to move into jobs. Lastly we look at what is involved in these jobs and the reality of the working life of a carer.

The health and social services are very much intertwined. Together they cover the **provision of care** and **support services**. We will be looking at jobs in the National Health Service, local authorities including education, the voluntary sector, and the private sector, and at informal care provided by the family and local community.

The National Health Service

The diagram opposite describes the areas of work in the National Health Service.

Areas of work In the National Health Service

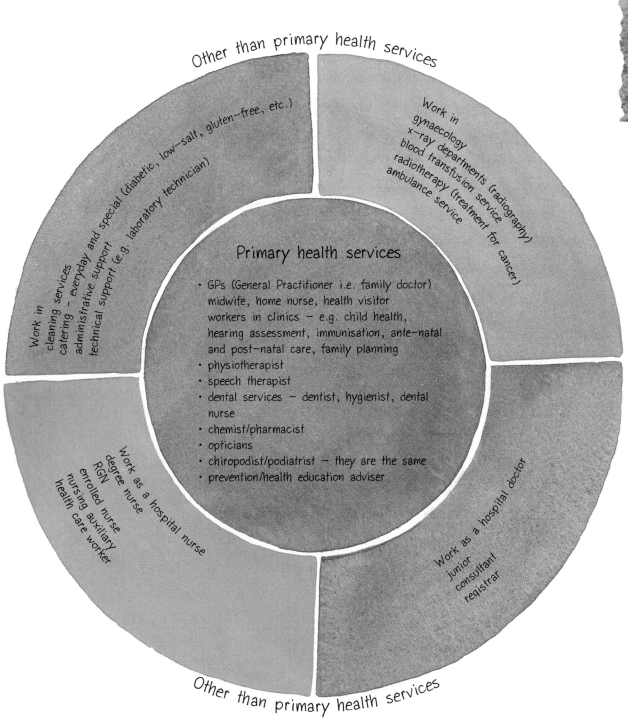

Other than primary health services

Work in
gynaecology
x-ray departments (radiography)
blood transfusion service
radiotherapy (treatment for cancer)
ambulance service

Work in
cleaning services
catering – everyday and special (diabetic, low-salt, gluten-free, etc.)
administrative support
technical support (e.g. laboratory technician)

Primary health services

- GPs (General Practitioner i.e. family doctor)
  midwife, home nurse, health visitor
  workers in clinics – e.g. child health,
  hearing assessment, immunisation, ante-natal
  and post-natal care, family planning
- physiotherapist
- speech therapist
- dental services – dentist, hygienist, dental nurse
- chemist/pharmacist
- opticians
- chiropodist/podiatrist – they are the same
- prevention/health education adviser

Work as a hospital nurse
degree nurse
RGN
enrolled nurse
nursing auxiliary
health care worker

Work as a hospital doctor
junior
consultant
registrar

Other than primary health services

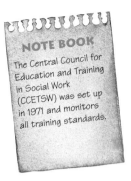

NOTE BOOK

The Central Council for Education and Training in Social Work (CCETSW) was set up in 1971 and monitors all training standards.

Local authorities

Social services

In the provision of social care, carers often work as

- caseworkers (with specific cases)
- fieldworkers (regularly working with specific clients)
- community workers (in the community with specific groups)

although these roles overlap.

Social workers can bring the statutory and voluntary services together to meet the immediate needs of people in times of crisis, and report in a practical way on how the services work together and with clients. The table below describes areas of work within the social services.

Areas of work in social services

Residential care
residential care worker
management of residential homes
registration and inspection of social care establishments
organising volunteers
statistics, publicity, etc.
expenditure control

Social work
social work services outside residential care
family placement of children needing care
court/school/police liaison
GP practice and hospital social workers
children – child protection, family work secure units etc.
services for disabled people – e.g. visually impaired
services for disadvantaged people – e.g. homeless
community work
translator, advocate

Domiciliary services
home help
day nurseries, day centres
aids and adaptations for disabled people to use at home
luncheon clubs
'Meals on Wheels'
adult training centres
rehabilitation centres i.e. helping people to become independent

Management
salaries and wages
recruitment
secretarial services
supplies
collecting contributions towards care where appropriate
burial arrangements (if there are no family or friends)
training, assessment, and provision

Areas of work in education

Education

Jobs	
teacher	caterer
classroom assistant (non-teaching)	cleaner
	gardener
technician	buildings
head teacher	supervisor/caretaker
bursar (looks after funds)	
secretarial work	
administration	

Age groups	Sector
nurseries	state, private, voluntary
infant/junior/primary	state, private, voluntary
secondary	state, private
further education	
higher education	all are independent of local authority control
adult education	

ACTIVITY A

1 Using the diagram and tables on pages 27 and 28, make a list of what you consider to be the main jobs in health and social care under the headings 'Direct Care' and 'Indirect Care'.

2 Discuss your decisions in a group and amend the list under the guidance of your tutor.

C2.1a

The voluntary sector

Examples of voluntary services providers include Dr Barnados, MIND, and The Samaritans. Most of their workers are volunteers and are unpaid. They may or may not be trained. Larger organisations need salaried staff with professional training to manage them.

Those who want to volunteer for work with a charitable organisation need to contact the Citizens' Advice Bureau or their local social services department. Training may or may not be part of the package. Sometimes a first aid qualification is required; sometimes, as in the area of counselling, specific training is demanded.

People's motives for working as volunteers are as varied as those of all carers. For some, a sense of duty or a religious commitment leads them to the work. Others see it as an antidote to the boredom of retirement or unemployment. Others have skills they want to share. Some use voluntary work to gain practical experience for paid occupation. There are those who wish to add weight to a pressure group for reform, and some who become involved out of sheer goodwill and gratitude for personal good fortune.

The private sector

The table below shows the type of services provided by carers in the private sector.

Areas of work in the private sector

Residential & day care	Child care	Health care	Other services
proprietor/owner/ manager	play groups – owner manager	occupational therapy	laundry
RGN (Registered General Nurse)	assistant	chiropody/podiatry	cleaning
enrolled nurse	holiday companies and tour operators	dentistry	hairdressing
care assistant	nanny	physiotherapy	nail care
respite care	childminder	alternative medicine	car hire
'sitting' schemes (relieving carers in their homes)	foster parent	homeopathy	reminiscence therapy
		reflexology	
		acupuncture	
		aromatherapy	
		chiropractic	
		osteopathy	

Informal care

Most health and social care is carried out by ordinary people within their families, or by specialist local groups.

One of the aims of the Community Care Act is that people should remain as independent as possible in their own homes. Thus the role of health and social care workers within the community has taken on a new and important significance. It is part of their role to work with informal carers and to link them with services which might make life easier for all concerned.

The day-to-day work of people with jobs in health and social care

In studying people's work in the health and social care field, we will be examining work patterns, working with client groups, and hours of work.

Work patterns

Work patterns vary within the areas of health and social care. The following list gives the main types of working patterns:

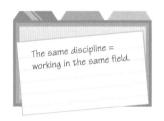

The same discipline = working in the same field.

- alone – childminders, foster parents

- in teams with the same discipline – a dental practice with a dentist, dental nurse, and hygienist

- in teams of people from various disciplines but with similar goals

  – GP's practice with a GP, practice nurse, community nurse, health visitor, chiropodist

  – community mental health team of social workers, community psychiatric nurse, clinical psychologist, community worker.

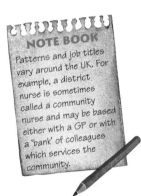

NOTE BOOK

Patterns and job titles vary around the UK. For example, a district nurse is sometimes called a community nurse and may be based either with a GP or with a 'bank' of colleagues which services the community.

Working with client groups

Those who have a close working relationship with clients can be regarded as being involved with treatment, enablement, or a combination of these two.

Treatment is the easier to define. It refers to the carer who is actively involved with caring for the physical or mental health of a client.

Enablement literally means making someone more able. Thus a social worker will make a client *more able* to be independent. A physiotherapist makes a client *more able* to move freely. An occupational therapist makes people *more able* to manipulate things and use their surroundings effectively.

Hours of work

Those working in the care services have work hours which vary greatly. Many workers are attracted by the unpredictability of the job and the irregular hours, feeling that they would find 'nine-to-five' work monotonous.

Some carers work during the day-time, others at night. This can be a matter of choice, or something imposed by the needs of clients. Both day and night work can be regular, or arranged into varying **shifts**.

Holiday time varies from job to job, but many carers work at Christmas and other times when many people are on holiday.

Career routes for people working in health and social care

Consideration of career routes needs to include study of qualifications, other entry requirements, previous jobs, possible future jobs, and opportunities for job relocation. These five aspects are covered together in the following text.

Entry qualifications for work in health and social care can be either **vocational** or **academic**.

Vocational qualifications, such as NVQs, first aid certificates, and work-based training, are

- practical, preparing for the world of work
- skills-based with background knowledge
- gained through training or work experience.

GNVQs are at present included in the vocational category – those at Advanced level are sometimes referred to as 'vocational A levels'.

Academic qualifications, such as GCSE, A levels, degrees, and diplomas, are

- knowledge-based
- gained through school/college/university, or by independent study linked to a college or university base.

When you are considering work in the field of health and social care or education, you need to decide how much you enjoy working close to people. If you like company, and relate well to others, you may choose a job which involves direct contact with clients. If you want to help society but are not enthusiastic about interacting with individuals needing care, you may prefer to go into the administrative, technical, or support side of health or social care.

National Vocational Qualifications (NVQs)

Until recently the majority of workers in the UK had no nationally recognised qualification. To put this right, NVQs were devised; they are awarded for skills and competence in a working situation.

The field of health and social care has been included in this revolutionary process. The NVQs in Care are designed for those working in residential and day care. The NVQs in Early Years Care and Education are for those looking after children up to seven years of age. There are NVQs in Operating Theatre Practice, Neurophysiology, Criminal Justice Services, Catering and Hospitality, and other areas in the field of health and social care.

The NVQs are primarily intended to reward **skills**, but, as they proceed up through the levels, the **knowledge content** becomes more significant.

General National Vocational Qualifications (GNVQs)

The GNVQs are, unlike the NVQs, knowledge-based, and are currently mainly gained in schools and colleges. Their method of assessment (by various ways of providing evidence) has evolved from the NVQ systems.

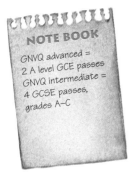

NOTE BOOK

GNVQ advanced =
2 A level GCE passes
GNVQ intermediate =
4 GCSE passes,
grades A–C

Routes to jobs

GNVQ Intermediate	Degree	Vocational
+ *NVQ* care assistant, health care worker, community care worker child care + *GNVQ Advanced* + *A Level* – nursing + *A level* – teaching *(varies according to locality)*	*via A level, GNVQ Advanced, or a mix of both* Junior doctor, registrar, GP, surgeon, consultant some nursing; general or psychiatric, midwifery, health visiting, specialist nurse social work administration dentistry teaching health promotion pharmacy management physiotherapy	some nursing; general or psychiatric, midwifery, health visiting, specialist nurse ambulance service cleaning services home help management nursing auxiliary health care worker community care worker care assistant classroom assistant secretarial work teaching

General notes on work in the care field

Routes to jobs are becoming more flexible, making change and progression easier. Mature employees often have their previous work experience taken into consideration. A woman who has been a classroom assistant while her family was young may find it easy to make a career change through teacher training if she meets the academic requirements. Or an experienced health care worker with a level 3 NVQ in Care may be accepted for nurse training if other requirements are also met.

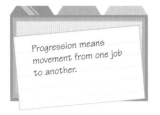

Progression means movement from one job to another.

Some jobs and qualifications give access to work throughout the UK, and others are more localised. Nurses are needed everywhere, while other work is clustered more in some areas than others. For instance, more social workers are needed in inner-city areas than rural ones.

Some jobs in care have a minimum age requirement. Social workers have to be 21.

The table on page 32 outlines the various routes to jobs in health and social care.

The realities of care work

Often the role of carers is romanticised. For example, Florence Nightingale is pictured gliding around darkened wards with her lamp, while adoring soldiers kiss her shadow. But, in reality, she was more likely to have had to tuck her skirts up to avoid the mud and slime, and the wards would have been full of dreadful smells, blood-soaked dressings, and emotionally scarred patients.

We need to examine the actualities of care work in a realistic way, realising that part of its attraction is that it is full of endless variety displayed by many different types of humanity.

unit one

Some everyday realities of care work

Pay (*approx*)

staff nurse £13–20,000 pa

sister £16–24,000 pa

health care assistant £8–10,000 pa

*care assistant £4.60–6.00 ph

ward secretary *from* £7,000 pa

social worker £14–21,000 pa

community care worker £7–9,000

education welfare officer £13–20,000 pa

dentist £22–50,000+ pa

dental nurse £4.45–5.65 ph

hygienist £13–18,000 pa

radiographer £13–15,000 pa

occupational therapist £14–16,000 pa

health service manager £15–50,000 pa

medical records clerk £8–9,000 pa

medical secretary *from* £9,000 pa

ambulance person *from* £11,000 pa

teacher £15–36,000 pa

school technician £7–10,000 pa

*classroom assistant £4.60–6.00 ph

pa = per annum   pw = per week   ph = per hour
*varies according to local rates
Source: Careers and Occupational Information Centre 1999

Main tasks

administration	feeding	giving medicines
report writing	family work	attending meetings
training others	counselling	advocacy
treatments	record keeping	telephoning
dressings	guidance	meeting the public
toileting	listening	liaising
washing		

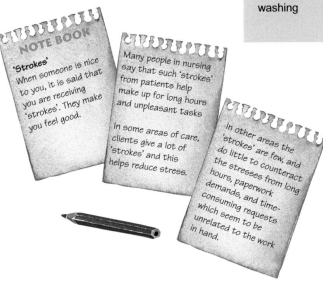

NOTE BOOK

'Strokes'
When someone is nice to you, it is said that you are receiving 'strokes'. They make you feel good.

Many people in nursing say that such 'strokes' from patients help make up for long hours and unpleasant tasks

In some areas of care, clients give a lot of 'strokes' and this helps reduce stress.

In other areas the 'strokes' are few, and do little to counteract the stresses from long hours, paperwork demands, and time-consuming requests which seem to be unrelated to the work in hand.

Working conditions

staff room

rest room

meal times

hours on standby

shifts/rotas

training possibilities

opportunities for travel

opportunities for career
  moves within the UK

'strokes'

resources

Work place

hospital ward

community

clinic

nursing homes

care homes

office

people's homes

community

schools

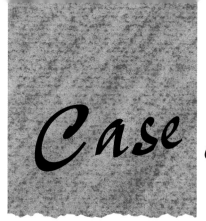

Case Studies

Task 1

1 Prepare a similar list of the work available in health, social care, and early years provision in your district.

2 Put the jobs into sector groups – NHS, local authority, voluntary, and private.

Case study 2.1   Netherfield Community Care

For some time, Debbie has had a vague ambition to become a 'social worker', but now she realises that it could be unrealistic for her to aim for a career requiring a degree, and decides to explore other avenues to community work. She asks Mikhail where she can find accurate, up-to-date information about jobs in health and social care in Netherfield. He brings her a list describing the various areas of work.

Case study 2.2   Hill Hall

In a tutorial session, the students are comparing notes about their work experience. Debbie and Ann are talking about their plans for the future. Ann, although she is now more accepting of the emotional stress of caring, still feels a bit nervous of tasks involving intimate and personal care of clients. But she dislikes the idea of routine office work, and wishes to commit herself to the care services. Debbie brings out Mikhail's list and shares it with the group. Together they work out jobs which Ann and others who share her feelings might undertake.

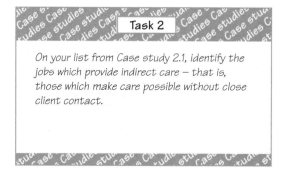

Task 2

On your list from Case study 2.1, identify the jobs which provide indirect care – that is, those which make care possible without close client contact.

Case study 2.3   The Thatched Cottage

Before he started working at The Thatched Cottage, Mark had wanted to go to a psychiatric hospital for his work experience, but he was too young. However, he now enjoys his placement. He expected it to be boring, but has found that he was mistaken. The residents have become real people to him. Their long lives have been so varied and interesting that their conversations are far from tedious. He likes the residents who are confused or demented most, as they come closest to his dream of working in mental health.

Task 3

1   How has Mark's idea of working in residential care for the elderly changed as he has become involved? What factors might have caused him to change his mind?

2   In what way will his experience be valuable if he pursues his ambition to be a mental health care worker?

Task 3

3   If Mark lived in your area, what choices would be open to him in the field of mental health?

4   What skills and qualifications would he need to take up each of the choices?

Record your conclusions in an appropriate format, using Key Skills in an imaginative way.

Case study 2.4   Down Way School

Adam is six. While he is talking to Jalwinder one day, he tells her that he believes that she, Isabel, and all the teaching staff live in the stock cupboard after school finishes each day. He thinks they stand up in line like clothes in a wardrobe. Jalwinder shares this in the staff room one rainy lunchtime, and, after the laughter dies down, the staff begin to discuss misunderstandings they used to hold about adults when they were little, especially about jobs.

Task 4

1   Think about three people known to your group who work as carers
   • one in indirect care
   • one in health and medical care
   • one in social care.
Working in a group, discuss and record what you think each job involves in terms of pay, working conditions, and tasks.

C2.1a, 2.2, 2.3

Task 4

2   Each word process a letter (including an address label) and send one copy to arrange a meeting with the three people concerned to find out

IT2.1, 2.2, 2.3

   • how your image of their work fits in with the reality of their job

Task 4

   • the skills and qualifications they needed before they started
   • if they would recommend their job to a young person starting work
   • whether or not they have received training
   • any ambitions they have for promotion or change of occupation.

Multiple Choice Questions

2.1 A career route is

   a *the way you decide to go to work*

   b *the requirements for entry into a job*

   c *a qualification gained at school or college*

   d *the beginning of work experience*

2.2 People who wish to take up social work must be

   a *over 18 years old*

   b *under 21 years old*

   c *over 21 years old*

   d *under 30 years old*

2.3 Which of the following phrases best describes an NVQ?

   a *a vocational award*

   b *a degree*

   c *a GNVQ*

   d *a diploma*

2.4 Which of the following is an example of a team of the same discipline?

   a *a classroom assistant, a care assistant, an enrolled nurse*

   b *a podiatrist (chiropodist), a health care worker, a nanny*

   c *a GP, a Trust hospital, a social worker*

   d *a dentist, a dental nurse, a hygienist*

2.5 Which of the following *best* describes shift work?

   a *taking turns to work for different periods of time*

   b *frequently moving from one job to another*

   c *working as part of a multi-disciplinary team*

   d *having to work with changing client groups*

2.6 Having opportunities for job relocation means

   a *working with a short-term contract*

   b *having to do night duty from time to time*

   c *following a flexible career route*

   d *having the choice to move to similar work elsewhere*

Note: These questions are for you to test your knowledge. There is no formal multiple choice test in this GNVQ.

Unit 1.3
Effective communication skills

After you have worked through this third section of Unit 1, you will understand why communication and interpersonal relationships need to be effective in health and social care.

You will be examining your own communication skills to see if they need to be developed to make your relationships with others more meaningful. Self-knowledge and self-evaluation are important for those hoping to work in services where people are in close contact with others.

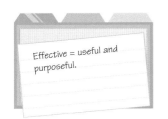

Effective = useful and purposeful.

Introduction

When we **communicate** we are in touch with another person or a group, and sharing, exchanging, or passing on information. From infancy to old age we communicate with the world around us – we may even talk to ourselves frequently!

Communication brings **power**. Good communicators can adjust what they say and how they say it to ensure that those receiving their information understand it. They subtly change their vocabulary, their accent, or their body language to make the listener feel at ease and more likely to hear what is being said.

Power brings **responsibility**. A carer who is a good communicator will use the power which follows to inform, encourage, reassure, and help clients. But good communication skills can be used irresponsibly – for example, when they are used to manipulate, bully, or intimidate other people.

We will be looking at the role of communication in the intellectual, emotional, and social development of the individual, in the formation of personal beliefs and preferences (including culture, religion, politics, sexuality), and in the development of groups.

Speaking and listening are difficult if there is anything wrong with the mouth, tongue, and vocal cords, or with the ears. Equally important is the state of development of the brain, where messages are received and understood. This is why children with physical disabilities may have problems with communication.

Development of self

Half of children's mental capacity will have developed before they are four. Learning is much faster if the child has language skills. Thoughts, feelings, ideas, and attitudes are easier to grasp through words. Reading extends our horizons. Discussion helps to form our ideas. Listening puts us in touch with other people's views. Thus our powers of communication extend our knowledge and help our intelligence to develop.

Intellectual development

Babies learn to speak as their muscles and systems develop and their understanding matures. In their pre-verbal stage babies cry, smile, gurgle, and make eye contact to communicate with their carers. Infants 'scribble talk' and babble and from 9 months they may say simple words.

Some people with learning difficulties or physical disabilities may never be able to speak clearly or use a wide vocabulary. If their eye–hand co-ordination is adequate they may be able to use a word board or a word processor, or point to pictures. Communication like this is slow and can lead to frustration unless the client is helped with patience and sensitivity. Many clients exceed everybody's predictions about their abilities if they are surrounded by encouraging and supportive carers.

Social and emotional development

As children grow up they learn to behave in a manner which is acceptable to the people around them. Their personalities usually develop within the family. Their responses to the family's behaviour determine how their emotions develop. Children whose social and emotional development has been hampered by social or emotional deprivations are often poor communicators.

Personal beliefs and preferences

As we grow and our ability to communicate by receiving and interpreting information develops, we begin to find out who we are, and to decide what our personal beliefs and preferences will be.

If someone has not had much contact with the outside world, individual choices may have been very narrow. This is why infant schools and nurseries try to provide as wide a spread of experiences as possible to children who may not have a range of possibilities at home. Carers often provide **guided choice**, which means that clients' choice is limited to, say, five options to avoid muddle and confusion.

To decide on personal beliefs and preferences people need to be able to exchange views and information about how they feel. Some people adopt their family's beliefs which have surrounded them since infancy. This is why culture and religious traditions survive for generations,

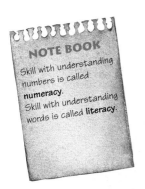

Communication boards have words or symbols on them, often in squares.

People who have difficulty in speaking point to the squares to help with communication.

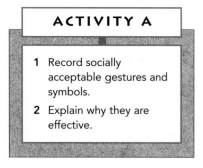

NOTE BOOK

Skill with understanding numbers is called **numeracy**.
Skill with understanding words is called **literacy**.

ACTIVITY A

1 Record socially acceptable gestures and symbols.

2 Explain why they are effective.

Autism is a condition in which the sufferer is unable to relate to people, and is often disturbed by change.

and why children may copy their parents' job choices and lifestyles. If children feel the need to turn their back on their family's ways, good communication with parents can make this a friendly experience, while without good communication family splits and hostilities may occur.

The social and emotional development of those with language and speech impairment is affected by teasing and mimicry, so that they feel rejected and isolated. People who are autistic do not appreciate jokes and high spirits, which is difficult for society to understand and causes them to feel rejected.

Young people especially like to talk to each other at great length, in school or college, at clubs and pubs. In adolescence, the foundations of adulthood are forming, so talking about things helps to consolidate feelings and ease anxieties. Lonely young people find this time especially hard if they have no friends in whom to confide about everything from family relationships through to politics and sexuality.

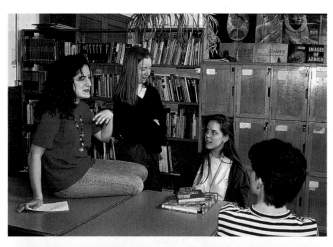

The social development of children with sensory impairment is often problematical. They find it hard to interpret other people's actions. Visually impaired people find it hard to learn by copying other people – a major factor in our social development – and cannot receive non-verbal messages like facial expressions and body language. They run the risk of offending by using inappropriate gestures, and will need to be taught socially acceptable ways of using non-verbal communications.

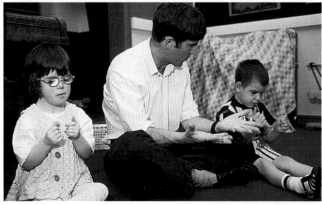

We acquire our concepts of the world mainly through spoken language. Hearing-impaired people find it hard to describe ideas or to understand feelings. They may appear to be slow learners, especially if their hearing problems are late in being identified, and their social development is often delayed as others find them hard to relate to, which in turn can cause difficulties with emotional development.

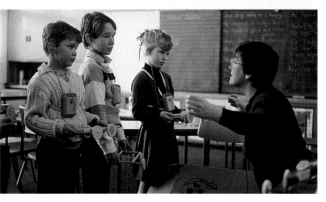

Development of groups and families

Communication plays an important part in the development of relationships.

The importance of communication to social interaction

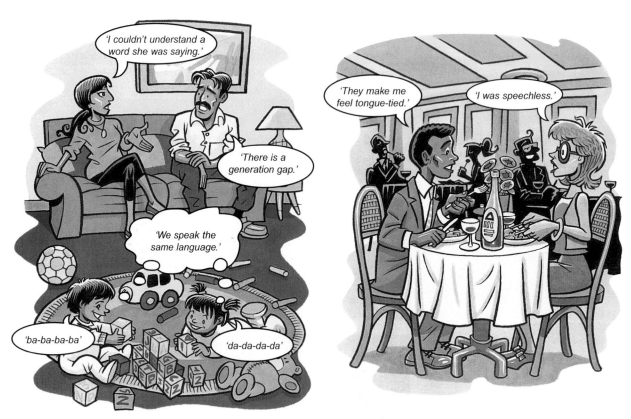

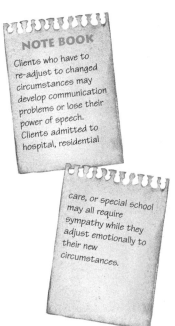

Communication with others is a basic human need. Children who have been actively encouraged to communicate find it natural to share experiences, co-operate with others, work out the results of their actions, make comparisons, and express their feelings. This gives them an advantage as emotionally secure adults, able to think and reason, understand and sympathise, and to share their ideas and feelings by effective communication.

Conversely, some clients have few of these advantages, and need to be persuaded and encouraged to share their true feelings so that they can be helped in the best possible way.

The language of emotions is rich, and uses rare words which may not be easily understood: words like 'distress', 'anxiety', 'foreboding', 'dread', 'depression', 'elation', 'apprehension', 'pain', 'excitement', 'pleasure', 'admiration', and 'hope'. When people's emotional vocabulary is limited to 'love', as in 'I love that song', or 'hate', as in 'I hate that food', it is hard for them to convey accurately how they feel when it really matters. They need practice before they can express exactly what their emotional needs are.

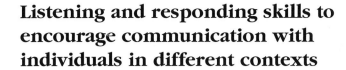

Listening and responding skills to encourage communication with individuals in different contexts

We communicate in many different ways. These include

- facial expression
- body language and eye contact
- sensory contact – that is, touch
- posture
- prompts, paraphrasing, and summarising
- asking open and closed questions
- the tone, pitch, and pace of our communication.

These seven methods are covered together in the text that follows.

Communicating effectively requires a combination of verbal and non-verbal methods. We may learn as much by looking as we do by listening, which is why some people prefer meeting face to face to speaking on the telephone. The table at the bottom of this page lists what you can do to help clients with language.

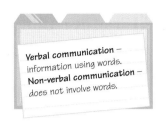

Verbal communication –
information using words.
Non-verbal communication –
does not involve words.

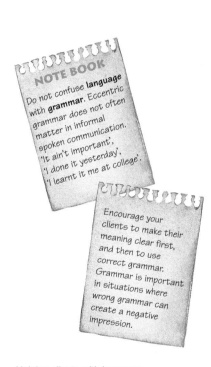

NOTE BOOK

Do not confuse language with **grammar**. Eccentric grammar does not often matter in informal spoken communication. 'It ain't important', 'I done it yesterday', 'I learnt it me at college'.

Encourage your clients to make their meaning clear first, and then to use correct grammar. Grammar is important in situations where wrong grammar can create a negative impression.

Appropriate facial expressions, body language, eye contact, and posture

We need to be careful about the message that our facial expressions and body language give to the person who is speaking to us. If we begin to show disapproval before someone has finished telling us something important, he or she could alter what is being said to fit what he or she has guessed we are thinking.

This often matters less in an informal situation than it does in a formal one, because when people feel relaxed enough to be totally honest with one another it is easier to put misunderstandings right later.

Helping clients with language

- Talk and listen, with much eye contact.
- Bathe clients in language. Give a running commentary about whatever you or they happen to be doing.
- Play/work together.
- Introduce many new experiences and objects.
- Read stories and watch and discuss TV programmes together.
- Give them books, even if reading is hard. Ensure the books are age-appropriate, not babyish, and match clients' interests, e.g. football, pop music.
- Go to the library together.
- Keep a scrap book.
- Use language that can be understood.
- Use pauses as a clue that it is the client's turn to speak.
- Show that you value their opinion.
- Play with blowing bubbles, and sucking a ping pong ball on a straw. (This will help with breath control, which aids speech.)
- Remember that it takes about a year of listening to a language before children can speak it.

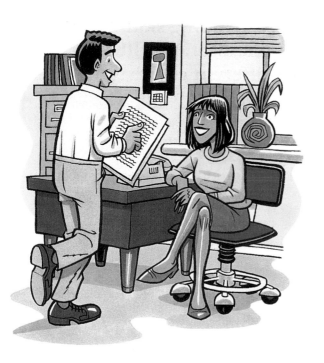

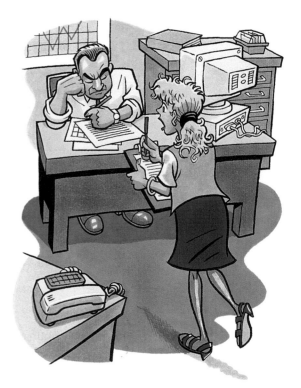

Eye contact implies interest and commitment. Use it even when you think that clients can neither see nor appreciate it – maybe because of impaired vision or confusion. Don't automatically expect eye contact from clients. They may be unaware of its importance or not interested in it, or unable to achieve it because of physical incapacity. Talk about the importance of eye contact to clients if it falls within your role in the workplace.

Posture

Most of what we communicate is conveyed in a way other than speech. Try lowering the volume on the television and see if you can guess what is going on from people's posture and body language. Think about pets. They manage to let us know a great deal without saying a word: 'I want feeding'; 'I want to go out'; 'I like being with you'; 'Welcome home'.

People give messages from the way they sit, stand, choose their seats in relation to one another, and move their hands, arms, and legs. Watch how people unconsciously copy each other. The gestures of the dominant person are often imitated. When listening to clients, carers need to make sure that what they say is matched with how it is being said. They need to behave in a way which shows interest, by nodding, turning towards the speaker, leaning forward a little, and sitting in a relaxed yet attentive way. The posture needs to be open, not with the arms folded and legs crossed.

It is important to pick up clues from clients to realise when they are feeling stressed or nervous, such as a tense position, a set expression, shallow breathing, a flushed or pale face, or fidgeting.

ACTIVITY B

Work out typical postures, body language, facial expressions, and eye contact indicating anger, impatience, fear, sympathy, interest, and concern.

You could use role play in this activity. Remember to record it in an appropriate way for your portfolio – maybe by video.

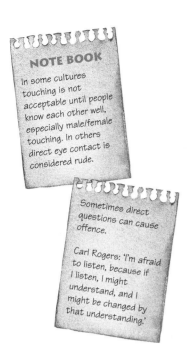

NOTE BOOK

In some cultures touching is not acceptable until people know each other well, especially male/female touching. In others direct eye contact is considered rude.

Sometimes direct questions can cause offence.

Carl Rogers: 'I'm afraid to listen, because if I listen, I might understand, and I might be changed by that understanding.'

Non-verbal messages are closely linked to acceptable behaviour in the society in which we live. Unlike words, posture and gesture have no fixed meanings and can be misinterpreted. In some societies it is considered unbecoming for a woman to look directly at a man. Smiling to show the teeth is thought to be very rude in some countries. Space is used in different ways. Many British people are most comfortable with a space between them of about two and half feet, and there is generally not much physical contact. Others stand closer together and touch one another more frequently.

Sensory contact

With **confused** people, touch can be misinterpreted as aggression. However, many clients are lonely. Elderly people may have lost a partner, be far from their family, and have had no physical contact for years. When you are sure that your meaning will not be misunderstood and that it is appropriate in the place of work, give your hugs and hand-holding freely, as a means of conveying warmth, sympathy, and a willingness to help.

Remember that some people object to being touched. You may need to touch gently people who have **hearing impairment**, in order to catch their attention.

Active listening

To listen actively, we need to concentrate so that we can pick out the points of what other people are saying and try to discover anything underlying the words which is a sign of what they may want to say but do not feel able to. You will get clues from

- facial expression
- body language and posture
- pauses and noises other than words
- tone of voice and pitch
- pace of conversation
- choice of words.

To do this you need to have distractions at a minimum, to be aware of your own prejudices and overcome them, and to be prepared to listen to things you may not want to hear.

The table on the left lists what you can do and what you should avoid doing for clear communication with clients.

When we have conversations, questions help to keep things moving. It is useful to develop skills in selecting the right sort of questions to encourage other people to be honest and not put up barriers between their thoughts and the person with whom they are speaking. This involves three main techniques: open questions, closed questions, and prompts.

Open questions

When you ask an **open question** it is like opening a door – this type of question invites a long and detailed answer, which will help you to understand a person's true meaning. Examples of open questions are:

Tips for clear communication

- Speak slowly, using words which are easily understood.
- Make sure people who lip-read can see your face – don't stand with the light behind you or cover your mouth with your hand.
- Sit down to talk to people in wheelchairs or in bed. Otherwise your body language is saying that you are more important than they are, or that you are anxious to get away.
- Do not talk about important or personal things in busy places. Go somewhere private.
- Seek other people's views.
- Listen actively.

- 'What's the matter?'

- 'How are you feeling today?'

- Little noises – 'hmm?' 'So?'

- 'How did you get on at the clinic yesterday?'

Closed questions

Asking a **closed question** is like closing a door – this type of question invites a short answer that may shut the conversation down, because it may only need a one-word answer. For example

- 'Tea or coffee?'

- 'Would you like a bath?'

- 'What's your name?'

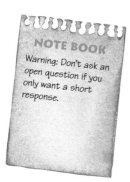

NOTE BOOK

Warning: Don't ask an open question if you only want a short response.

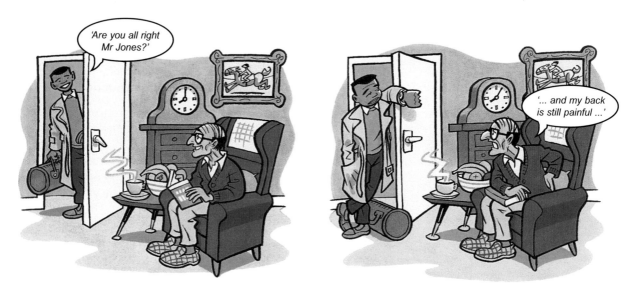

Answer takes five minutes.

or

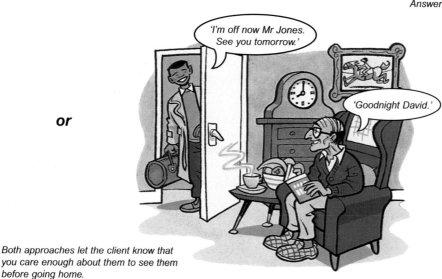

Both approaches let the client know that you care enough about them to see them before going home.

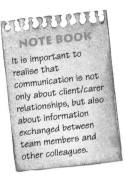

NOTE BOOK

It is important to realise that communication is not only about client/carer relationships, but also about information exchanged between team members and other colleagues.

unit one

Prompts

Prompts give clues to possible answers. They serve to keep the conversation going. For example

- 'Did you like that?'
- 'Was it difficult?'

Paraphrasing and summarising

We clarify what we think we have heard and understood by statements beginning

- 'Am I right in thinking that you . . . ?'
- 'Do you mean that . . . ?'

This gives the person being spoken to the opportunity to correct any misinterpretation and shows that you have been listening and therefore that you care.

Tone, pitch, and pace of communication

When talking to a client, you need to consider the impact of your

- **tone** – for example, loud, angry, or sympathetic
- **style** – for example, simple and clear for young children, or using longer and more complicated sentences for a more mature person
- **pace** – fast or slow.

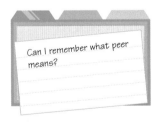

Can I remember what peer means?

ACTIVITY C

Can you think of an occasion when you have modified your verbal or non-verbal behaviour or your appearance to make it more suitable to the people you are with?

Write a short account of it.

C2.3

Observation skills to encourage communication in different contexts

We will be exploring the fact that people change their verbal behaviour, non-verbal behaviour, and appearance according to the **context** they are in. For example, a person may be in a one-to-one situation, in a group of three or more, with a peer group, or in a group including people of different status.

Sometimes behaviour needs to be changed or adjusted because it is not appropriate to the context. Care workers need to be aware of this so that they can take careful notice of their own and other people's behaviour and modify it if necessary.

The care worker may need to suggest that a client should modify his or her behaviour. Adults who have **learning difficulties** may be loving and affectionate by nature. It seems a pity to discourage them from showing affection, but part of the **normalisation** process is to encourage them to behave in an **age-appropriate** manner. Thus we try to teach them that most adults do not kiss the bus driver or cuddle someone to whom they have just been introduced. Allowing such behaviour to continue sets clients up as objects of ridicule, and is not fair to them.

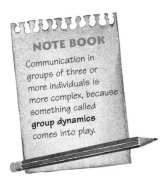

When we communicate with only one other person, an onlooker can immediately tell our relationship by our non-verbal communication. This reflects whether we are with a friend, an acquaintance, a stranger, or someone whom we feel is less or more important than us.

ACTIVITY D

Thinking about how you behave with a friend, an acquaintance, a stranger, and someone whom you feel is less or more important than yourself, work out how your behaviour changes in terms of

- verbal behaviour
- non-verbal behaviour
- appearance.

ACTIVITY E

1 Imagine you are watching a small group of people

   a at a bus stop   **b** in a café   **c** at a meeting.

What in their verbal behaviour, non-verbal behaviour, and appearance would tell you whether they are friends, work colleagues, or employers and employees?

2 Record your conclusions.

Obstacles to effective communication

Many things prevent people from understanding one another. They fall into two categories: environmental obstacles and social and cultural constraints.

Environmental obstacles

The following environmental obstacles prevent effective communication:

- distractions – e.g. the television being on, and other noises
- aids not working or missing – spectacles, hearing aid, badly fitted false teeth, communication board, pen and pencil
- impatience – no time allowed for answers or thinking space
- misinterpreting words and gestures
- communicating when the client is tired
- acute infection/illness causing confusion and temporary loss of understanding

- lack of concentration
- boredom
- inappropriate lighting.

Social constraints

It would be nice to think that people felt truly equal to each other. As soon as one feels either superior or inferior to another, problems in communicating begin. This may be given away by either their verbal or their non-verbal communication. The messages can be summed up in the expressions

'I'm OK. You're OK.'   (*equal* relationship)

'I'm OK. You're not OK.'
'I'm not OK. You're OK.' } (*unequal* relationship)

ACTIVITY F

For this activity you will work with someone who is **of a different status from yourself**. Before you begin, work out with your colleagues what this means. With this person

1 Discuss the significance of the statement of equality 'I'm OK. You're OK' in the context of communication and interpersonal skills. **C2.1, 2.3**

2 Work out how being with someone felt to be

   a more important than oneself

   b less important than oneself

   may be an obstacle to effective communication.

3 Record your observations in an appropriate way. **IT2.1, 2.2, 2.3**

Cultural constraints

The main and most obvious barrier is a language one, but non-verbal communication can cause unintentional offence. In this country we are used to plenty of personal space. We don't stand too close together, we are not particularly demonstrative (that is, we don't show emotion), and we may be brought up not to share our feelings. These can all be misinterpreted by people of other cultures, and vice versa. The box on the left shows how one characteristic can be seen as a completely different characteristic by another person/culture.

People's views of people

interested	nosy
polite	cold
enthusiastic	pushy
warm	clinging
affectionate	demanding
articulate	egghead
chatty	noisy

We need to appreciate the deep differences between cultures so that we do not offend unintentionally and cause others to treat us so warily that true communication becomes impossible.

Language

Sometimes we use inappropriate words, give too much information at once, or speak too fast. This is an important consideration when

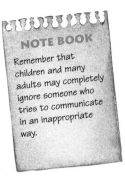

NOTE BOOK

Remember that children and many adults may completely ignore someone who tries to communicate in an inappropriate way.

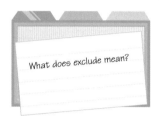

What does exclude mean?

working with clients who themselves have a limited vocabulary, who do not speak English fluently, or who have impaired hearing.

Before being totally accepted into a new group, individuals have to undergo a learning process during which they learn the special words and **jargon** of the group. This is more marked when a language other than the native one is involved, such as when people of different nationalities marry and need to communicate with members of one another's extended family. Groups develop jargon, either at work or socially. This excludes those outside the group.

ACTIVITY G

1 Make a list of jargon words.
2 Record which groups will understand these words, and which groups will be excluded by not understanding them.

Physical or intellectual constraints

Confused or demented people often respond readily to non-verbal communication and are surprisingly good at picking up messages that the carer had thought had been well hidden like: 'I'm frightened of you'.

Communication impairment

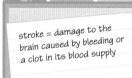

stroke = damage to the brain caused by bleeding or a clot in its blood supply

Autism
• impaired understanding of the meaning of language and social situations
• cannot sympathise with other people's feelings and have few natural social skills
• need to be taught how to behave
• may become excessively anxious when things go wrong
• may not respond warmly or affectionately (which does not mean that we should not respond warmly or affectionately)

Dysarthria
• nerve supply is disrupted, making speech slurred – e.g. after a stroke
• understanding and desire to speak are not affected

Dysphasia
• loss of ability to use words properly – e.g. after a stroke nouns are commonly lost and the client may use words like 'thingummyjig' to fill the gaps.
• sometimes use similar-sounding words wrongly – e.g. 'lock' for 'clock', 'mess' for 'dress'.
• may nod and say 'no' when they mean 'yes'.
• carers need to listen for the meaning and not to the words.

Inappropriate language
• some clients with communication problems pepper their speech with recurrent words. These may be quite rude swear words, or phrases like 'I wonder, I wonder, I wonder', with no meaning in the normal sense.

Evaluation of one's own communication skills and suggestions for their improvement

Good communication is an art which can be learned. Some people seem to have been born good communicators, but it is more likely that they have been allowed and enabled to develop good communication skills during their upbringing and schooling.

In order to improve as communicators, we need to be able to work out how good we are already and where improvements are needed. There are three stages to this type of evaluation, involving self-appraisal, feedback from others, and improvement in methods and techniques.

You have spent time looking at what helps and what hinders communication. In activities H, I, J, and K, you will have a chance to work with what you have learnt.

Note: Remember to be gentle with each other's feelings during these activities. They are a test of your communication skills. If they become destructive instead of being useful, you will have to re-examine the effectiveness of communications within your group.

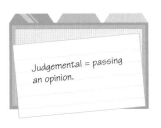

Judgemental = passing an opinion.

ACTIVITY H

Self-appraisal

Before you go on to find out how you appear to others as a communicator, answer yes or no to the following.

A When you talk, do you:

1 maintain eye contact without staring

2 assume other people feel the same as you do about things

3 talk more than you listen

4 use irritating language, such as jargon, slang, or swear words

5 forget that the way you communicate carries messages about the sort of person you are

6 mumble or whisper

7 make sure your listener understands what you are trying to say

8 try to use words that the listener will understand?

To be a good communicator you should answer yes to questions 1, 7, 8 and no to questions 2, 3, 4, 5, 6.

B When you listen do you:

1 jump to conclusions

2 ask for clarification

3 change the subject

4 respond in the right way – for example, being serious when you are being told something important

5 interrupt

6 avoid being judgemental

7 think of your next question, not what is being said

8 react sympathetically instead of feeling threatened

9 pick up little things rather than important ones

10 co-operate rather than compete

11 pretend to understand

12 switch off?

To be a good communicator you should answer yes to questions 2, 4, 6, 8, 10 and no to questions 1, 3, 5, 7, 9, 11, 12.

ACTIVITY 1

Feedback from others

Select one of the following topics for discussion:

- What I would do if I won the National Lottery.
- What I like about my friends.
- My hobby.
- The time I was most scared.
- Where I would like to live.

Spend five minutes preparing your topic.

Work in groups of three – a speaker, a listener, and an observer.

The speaker tells the listener about the chosen topic, while the listener seeks to understand as much as possible at the same time.

Spend five minutes on this.

The observer gives a five-minute feedback on what has been seen or heard to help or hinder communication between the two, using the checklist below.

All three in the group will take turns to be the speaker, the listener, and the observer.

Read through the checklist before you start. Record your responses – maybe by video.

CHECKLIST

Speaker	Listener
prepared what was going to be said	didn't take over
clarity of speech	was sympathetic
tone of voice	didn't interrupt
appropriate choice of words	eye contact
eye contact	faced the speaker
logical order of ideas	asked relevant questions
pauses for questions	seemed interested
attitude – friendly	summarised at the end
verbal and non-verbal communication gave the same message	good body language – didn't fidget or look bored
	verbal and non-verbal communication gave the same message

Did the speaker behave in a normal way?

Did the listener behave in a normal way for him or her?

Are there ever barriers to effective listening in his or her everyday life?

1 Present a comparison, in the form of a pie chart, of the different ways in which you would spend money won on the National Lottery – e.g. on clothes, leisure, holidays, electronic equipment.

N2.1, 2.2, 2.3

2 Collect information about different people's hobbies and present the information in the form of a pie chart and bar chart to stimulate discussion within the group.

3 Collect information about different fears and then categorise before presenting in an appropriate way. Bring in percentages.

4 Collect information about where a group of people would like to live. Express in an appropriate form.

5 Enter these tasks on a spreadsheet and produce the charts and information required using a computer.

IT2.1, 2.2, 2.3

ACTIVITY J

Improvement in techniques

Think about

- open questions
- closed questions
- prompts.

List three examples of each that you used or could have used during Activity I (page 50) or during some other recent activity. List three examples of each that other people have used when talking to you recently. Complete the following table.

How I feel about asking:	
open questions	
closed questions	
probes	
prompts	

1 = not confident   **2** = fairly confident   **3** = confident

ACTIVITY K

Improvement in methods

Using your findings from Activities I and J, work out how you score in the communication methods shown in the table on the right. Work in pairs.

◀▶ Extension opportunity

As members of the group receive a score for each part of the communication section, work out mode, median, and mean score

a for each individual

b for the group.

Discuss the most appropriate form of average to use when choosing a value representative of the group.

Now you know what you need to change.

Methods of verbal and non-verbal communication

Use a scale of **1–5**:   **1** = room for improvements, **2** = not bad, **3** = effective,
4 = very good, **5** = excellent.

Verbal communication methods	1	2	3	4	5
Spoken					
• appropriate level of language					
• appropriate choice of words					
• amount of jargon					
• amount of slang					
• number of swear words					
Written					
• legibility of writing					
• ability to express thoughts					
Non-verbal communication methods					
Tone of voice					
Eye contact					
Facial expression					
Touch/physical contact					
Gestures					
Mime/sign language*					
Body language					
Use of personal space					
Dress/image					
'I'm OK/you're OK' messages					

* delete if not appropriate

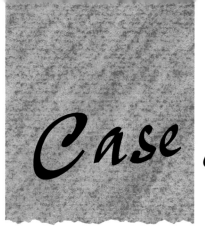

Case Studies

Case study 3.1   Hill Hall

Ann is rather frightened of Aamon, one of the older children who has a tendency to aggressive behaviour. She likes to keep an eye on him all the time, so she always leaves the door open when toileting him, but this appears to cause him to have outbreaks of temper. Aamon has limited speech, but can communicate with those who have time to persevere.

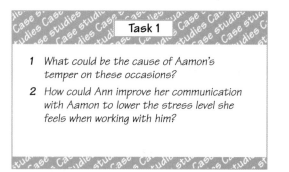

Task 1

1   What could be the cause of Aamon's temper on these occasions?

2   How could Ann improve her communication with Aamon to lower the stress level she feels when working with him?

Case study 3.2   Netherfield Community Care

Mr Dobzanski is a client who is rather fond of Debbie, and she becomes very embarrassed when he starts writing notes to her – 'Debbie means beaty', 'I beleaive in love' etc. She doesn't know how to respond, yet knows she must keep visiting him as part of her duties. She asks Mikhail to help, as she is afraid that Mr Dobzanski will not understand that his attentions are unwelcome, and may assume that she is mocking his poor spelling. He is very sensitive, and Debbie is keen not to offend him.

Mikhail and Debbie need to

1   let Mr Dobzanski know that his behaviour is inappropriate

2   do this without damaging his self-esteem

3   explain to him that they are acknowledging his emotional needs at the same time as Debbie's.

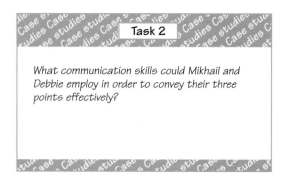

Task 2

What communication skills could Mikhail and Debbie employ in order to convey their three points effectively?

Case study 3.3   Down Way School

One day there is a great row in the corridor outside the classroom where Jalwinder is working. A father is threatening loudly to take a baseball bat to his daughter if she doesn't do what the headteacher wants her to do. The head is trying to persuade him to go into her room. All the children are listening with their mouths open, and one of them begins to cry. There are two communication issues here, one between the head and the father, and another between the classroom staff and the children.

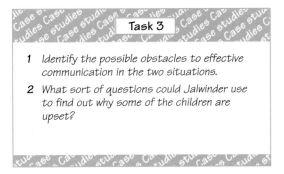

Task 3

1   Identify the possible obstacles to effective communication in the two situations.

2   What sort of questions could Jalwinder use to find out why some of the children are upset?

Case study 3.4   The Thatched Cottage

It is a big day for Dora. She is going to be assessed for several units of her NVQ by a visiting assessor. Later she tells Mark about it over a cup of tea. She says it was awful. She was nervous, and the assessor was very posh and made her feel stupid. She couldn't understand the feedback on her performance. The client they were working with had been really difficult and refused to let Dora put her teeth in. Despite having been successful, Dora is quite upset by the experience. She herself is going to assess Mark for an NVQ element, and promises him that she has learnt a lot about how not to behave when assessing someone.

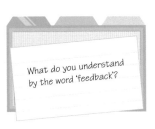

What do you understand by the word 'feedback'?

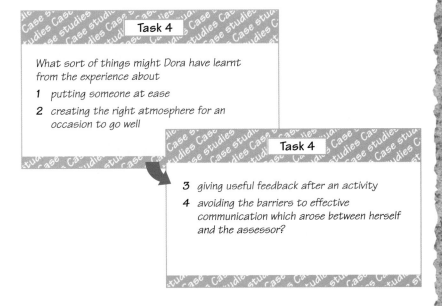

Task 4

What sort of things might Dora have learnt from the experience about

1   putting someone at ease

2   creating the right atmosphere for an occasion to go well

Task 4

3   giving useful feedback after an activity

4   avoiding the barriers to effective communication which arose between herself and the assessor?

Multiple Choice Questions

3.1 Which of the following is an example of an open question?

    a *'Did you manage well?'*

    b *'How did you manage after that had happened?'*

    c *'You managed well, did you?'*

    d *'After that, you managed all right, didn't you?'*

3.2 Self-appraisal and feedback are methods of

    a *interpretation*

    b *interaction*

    c *evolution*

    d *evaluation*

3.3 An unsuitable environment and language misunderstandings are

    a *useful to communication*

    b *obstacles to communication*

    c *methods of communication*

    d *contexts for communication*

3.4 Which one of the following is a communication skill?

    a *environment*

    b *evaluation*

    c *suitable facial expression*

    d *peer group pressure*

3.5 Which of the following is an important reason for developing communication skills?

    a *to acknowledge people's beliefs and preferences*

    b *to allow carers to manipulate clients*

    c *for self-appraisal*

    d *to overcome cultural constraints*

3.6 Verbal communication means

    a *using body language*

    b *listening to people*

    c *speaking to people*

    d *using touch*

Note: These questions are for you to test your knowledge. There is no formal multiple choice test in this GNVQ.

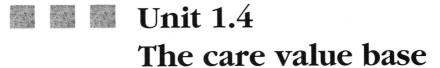

Unit 1.4
The care value base

The care value base underlies the whole of work in health, social care, and early years services. It includes anti-discriminatory practice, maintaining confidentiality of information, promoting individuals' rights to dignity, independence, health and safety, acknowledging their personal beliefs and identity, and finding imaginative ways of supporting them if ordinary approaches don't work.

Anti-discriminatory practice

Discrimination means treating people differently, or making distinctions between them. Unfair discriminatory behaviour affects relationships between individuals and groups in a damaging way.

The first part of Unit 1.4 examines the theories and concepts of unfair discrimination, looking at the forms that such discrimination may take, behaviour indicating discrimination, and the effects of discrimination.

The forms discrimination may take

We will be looking at seven areas which are the common bases for discrimination:

1 age
2 disability
3 gender
4 health status
5 race
6 religion
7 sexuality.

Age

Individuals are often labelled by their age. Children and young people are sometimes singled out for particular treatment. For example, the following measures are intended to protect young people during their development, and therefore these are not discriminatory practices.

- Young people are excluded from places where alcohol is served.
- Young people are not eligible to vote until the age of eighteen.
- It is illegal to sell cigarettes to young people.
- They are excluded from certain forms of employment until a minimum age is reached.

However, speaking in a patronising manner to children and young people, or ignoring them, are forms of discrimination indicating that they are not being treated as worthwhile individuals.

In a similar way, older people are discriminated against when they are treated disrespectfully by others younger than themselves. Some jobs are closed to people in late middle age. In their old age people are sometimes treated like pets or rather large infants.

Disability

Care workers of a generation ago tell how disabled members of families were sometimes kept in a shed at the bottom of the garden with their meals taken down to them. The only work available to them was that which could be undertaken in the shed.

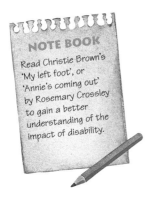

NOTE BOOK

Read Christie Brown's 'My left foot', or 'Annie's coming out' by Rosemary Crossley to gain a better understanding of the impact of disability.

Things have improved since then, but still people with physical disabilities are often excluded from jobs in which they could use their intelligence and knowledge despite their handicaps. People with learning disabilities, especially where these are severe, are, sadly, still sometimes treated with little respect.

Consider the options for people who are visually impaired, deaf, or in a wheelchair, or who have cerebral palsy, autism, or Down's syndrome.

Gender

Men and women are not always treated as equal. This sometimes happens within certain cultural groups where men are seen as socially superior to women. Some years ago women were said to be disadvantaged in education. The current trend is for girls to achieve better GCSE results than boys at 16 years old. The number of women gaining degrees and returning to education as mature students also appears to be increasing proportionately more quickly than the number of men.

In the field of care, most workers are women, and so it is easy to forget that women can be discriminated against in employment. In health care it is men who have to prove themselves as care assistants, midwives, nurses, and health care workers, in the same way that women have to in, say, the world of engineering or the fire service.

As single parents, who are most often women, are seen to be bringing children up successfully, young men may begin to feel inadequate. They may lack male role models, especially if they attend a school with mainly female teachers.

Traditionally women in our society remain the main carers. They are expected to look after elderly relatives, maybe sacrificing their chance of marriage to do so. It is far less common for men to take on this role.

Health status

The following table includes some examples of groups whose health problems may cause them to be discriminated against.

In the area of mental health
- people with schizophrenia
- people who suffer from depression
- people with behavioural problems

In the area of physical health
- people with epilepsy
- people who have AIDS or are HIV-positive
- people who have an ileostomy or colostomy

In a range of categories
- people who are homeless
- drug abusers
- people with alcohol-related problems
- those who have been in prison
- travelling families

Groups of people who may experience discrimination

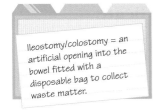

Ileostomy/colostomy = an artificial opening into the bowel fitted with a disposable bag to collect waste matter.

Race

Race, culture, and ethnic origin are closely linked. **Race** is to do with people's physical characteristics, for example the colour of their skin and eyes, the shape of their faces, or hair characteristics.

Ethnicity, ethnic origin, and **culture** determine which clothes people wear, their behaviour with each other, what they eat, and the language they use. An **ethnic minority** is a cultural group not widely represented in the area in which its people live.

Religion

Religion crosses race and cultural boundaries. Six of the main world religions are Buddhism, Christianity, Hinduism, Islam (practised by Muslims), Judaism, and Sikhism. Sadly, many of the worst wars are fought in the name of religion, even between sects of the same religion.

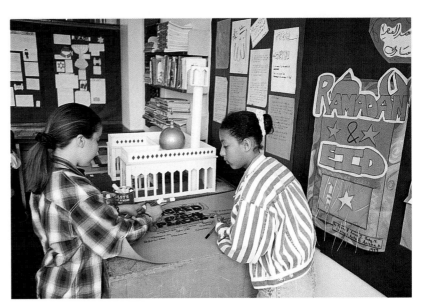

Countries with a rich and diverse history, such as the United Kingdom and the USA, have people of many races and cultures living together. They are said to be **multi-racial** and **multi-cultural** societies.

It is discriminatory not to allow a person or group to practise their cultural beliefs in a way appropriate to them, or not to provide food acceptable to them when they are in a care setting.

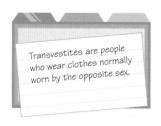

Transvestites are people who wear clothes normally worn by the opposite sex.

Sexuality

Examples of groups who may be discriminated against in our society include homosexual men, lesbians, and transvestites.

People's sexuality is a private matter. It may be complicated and unusual, and there is no reason why it should be made public. It is only when it breaks the law that it needs to be discussed with others.

Carers are in a privileged position in that they often hear clients' most personal secrets. They are also vulnerable, as they may discover something which they personally find distasteful. The boundaries of confidentiality are explored later.

Behaviours which may indicate discrimination

Discrimination may be **direct** or **indirect**.

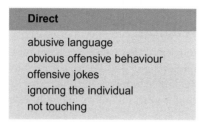
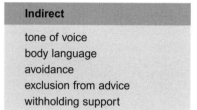

Direct	Indirect
abusive language	tone of voice
obvious offensive behaviour	body language
offensive jokes	avoidance
ignoring the individual	exclusion from advice
not touching	withholding support

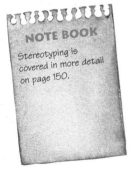

NOTE BOOK
Stereotyping is covered in more detail on page 150.

Direct discriminatory behaviour

Abusive language

People whose appearance makes them stand out may be subjected to abusive language. Racial groups, people with obvious disabilities, and those who dress differently from the majority are particularly likely to suffer in this way.

Verbal abuse is often a result of extreme stereotyping. It may show that the person being abused is considered to be of inferior status and seen to be lacking the power to retaliate. Abusive language is a form of emotional abuse. It is not always obvious, and whispers can be very sinister. Mockery, put-downs, and name-calling are all examples of abusive language.

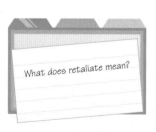

What does retaliate mean?

Obvious offensive behaviour

The word used for this is **overt**, which means it can be seen. The opposite is **covert**, which means it is hidden. Overt offensive behaviour ranges from pushing or spitting to causing physical harm, such as in attacks with a racist motive or against homosexuals.

Children and old people are sometimes treated roughly. Men and women are sometimes subjected to offensive behaviour which amounts to sexual harassment.

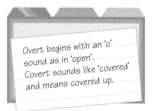

Overt begins with an 'o' sound as in 'open'.
Covert sounds like 'covered' and means covered up.

Sexual abuse is an extreme form of overt offensive behaviour. It can occur for discriminatory reasons, to enforce power, to humiliate, or for gratification with someone who cannot protect himself or herself and who is regarded therefore as being inferior.

Racist or sexist jokes

It is often those who feel most threatened who feel the need to make racist or sexist jokes. Although people who object to such jokes may be accused of lacking a sense of humour, they are right to object, as these jokes reinforce race or sex stereotypes in a harmful way.

Ignoring

We are offended if a shop assistant carries on a private conversation while we wait to be served. It makes us feel small. Likewise, clients feel excluded if two carers chat over their heads without including them in their conversation.

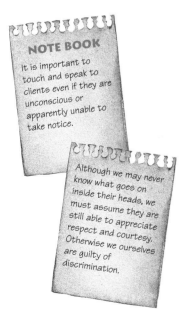

NOTE BOOK

It is important to touch and speak to clients even if they are unconscious or apparently unable to take notice.

Although we may never know what goes on inside their heads, we must assume they are still able to appreciate respect and courtesy. Otherwise we ourselves are guilty of discrimination.

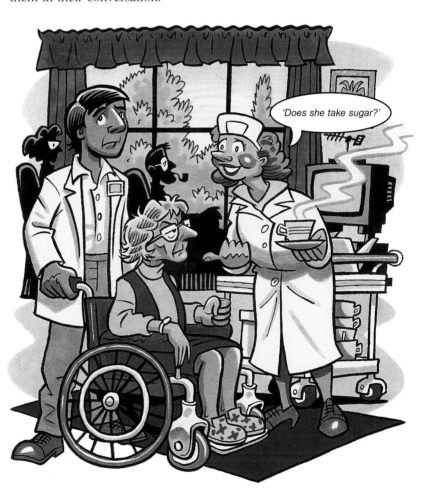

'Does she take sugar?'

Not touching

Lepers used to ring a bell to warn people they were coming so that they could be avoided. Today, if we withhold touch from someone, we are denying them their social acceptability in a similar way.

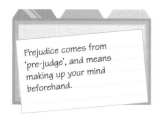

Prejudice comes from 'pre-judge', and means making up your mind beforehand.

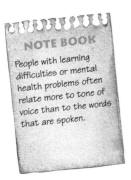

NOTE BOOK

People with learning difficulties or mental health problems often relate more to tone of voice than to the words that are spoken.

How our body language speaks

Some groups of people who may be avoided because of prejudice are

- those who are HIV-positive
- those who have skin complaints
- those of a different race or culture
- elderly people
- people who are incontinent
- people who are deformed or seen as ugly.

Indirect discriminatory behaviour

Tone of voice

It can be discriminatory to sound patronising, sneering, disapproving, suggestive, angry, or sarcastic. We can express all these feelings not by our choice of words but by the tone in which we speak. Likewise, when you hear a foreign language it is easy to guess the mood of the conversation by the tone of voice used by the speakers.

Body language

If a person is not to feel rejected, our body language needs to make them feel accepted. The following tables give examples of body language that expresses rejecting and accepting.

Ways to reject	Ways to accept
avoiding eye contact	making eye contact
arms folded	relaxing the hands and shoulders
standing at a distance	not standing too far away
leaning over a person	sitting down next to someone in a wheelchair or in a bed
not smiling	smiling
hands on hips	

Avoidance

People who have had a dreadful personal misfortune, such as the death of a loved one or bad news of severe illness, report that their friends sometimes cross the road to avoid speaking to them. This is very hurtful. When it is done from discriminatory motives it is extremely insulting.

Exclusion from advice

Recently a black woman, who was overweight to a degree which was life-threatening, stated that she was offered no health care advice to encourage her to lose weight. It was not until she found a doctor from her own ethnic background that she received information which was realistic and understandable.

A small number of elderly people in the UK have AIDS. They complain that no support is appropriate for them; all AIDS literature is aimed at young people.

When someone speaks English fairly fluently, but not as their first language, it may not be obvious if they do not understand everything that is said. Advice may be denied to people because they cannot read, cannot read English, or have difficulty understanding if the information is not presented in a pictorial or simple style.

Young adults with learning disabilities need access to health promotion advice and support with regard to their sexuality. To assume that they don't is to deny them their rights.

An example of direct discrimination	**An example of indirect discrimination**
An Asian person is not offered a job because he or she is Asian.	An employer devises a test which is culturally biased so that an Asian candidate is likely to fail.

The possible effects of discrimination

When people experience discrimination, the results are negative and harmful. The effects of this can be short-term or long-term, in which case they can be much more serious.

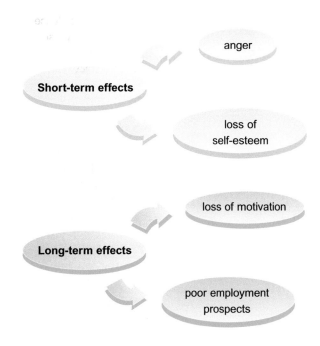

61

Short-term effects

Anger

Anger can act as a positive or negative force. Sometimes anger is directed into self-improvement, but more usually it is used to destroy material things – such as property, gardens, and cars – or abstract things – like relationships, self-image, and opportunities.

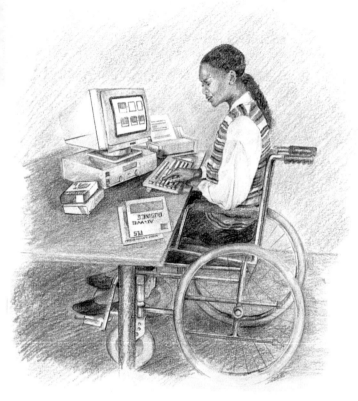

Determined anger (assertive behaviour):
'I'll show them what I'm capable of!'

Destructive anger (aggressive behaviour):
'I'll show them.'

Loss of self-esteem (self-worth)

Everybody can understand loss of self-esteem, so it is within all of us to be able to sympathise with how people experiencing discrimination must feel for much of the time. We may all experience it occasionally. For many it is a permanent state.

ACTIVITY A

Discuss how people's self-concept will be affected when they are unable to find meaningful employment because of discrimination on **three** of these bases.

- age/youth
- race
- disability
- gender
- health status.

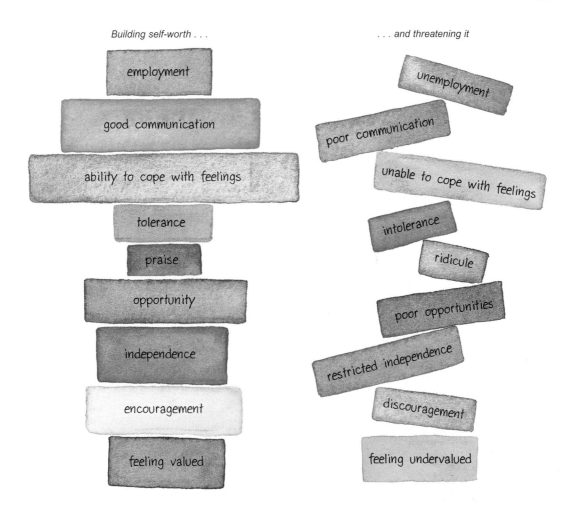

Building self-worth . . .

- employment
- good communication
- ability to cope with feelings
- tolerance
- praise
- opportunity
- independence
- encouragement
- feeling valued

. . . and threatening it

- unemployment
- poor communication
- unable to cope with feelings
- intolerance
- ridicule
- poor opportunities
- restricted independence
- discouragement
- feeling undervalued

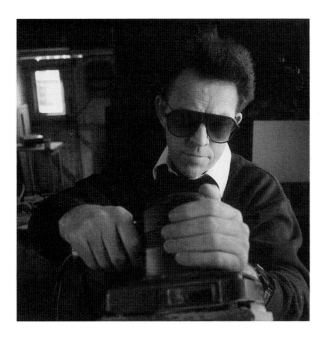

Long-term effects

Detrimental employment prospects

Stereotyped attitudes are self-confirming. If poorly paid jobs, which most of society does not want to do, are the only ones in which people of certain groups manage to gain employment, then it is easy to form the opinion that those are the only jobs they are able to do. Ultimately such employees may become resigned to thinking they are capable of nothing better, when in reality they may have other talents worthy of being developed if the opportunity arose.

His visual impairment has not prevented this man from developing craft skills.

Driving forces

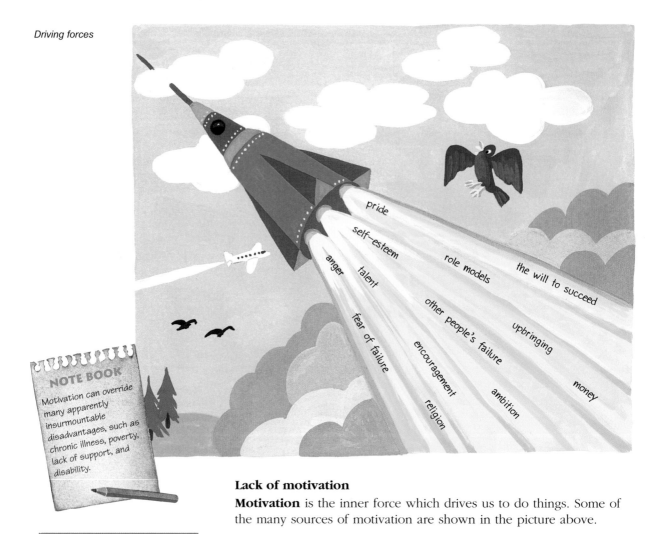

NOTE BOOK
Motivation can override many apparently insurmountable disadvantages, such as chronic illness, poverty, lack of support, and disability.

Lack of motivation
Motivation is the inner force which drives us to do things. Some of the many sources of motivation are shown in the picture above.

ACTIVITY B

1 The diagram on the right shows a list of motivational forces. Work out and then mark on the diagram whether these forces may work for (use a tick '✔') or against (use a cross '✗') groups who are discriminated against.

Taking into consideration the different sources of motivation, conduct a survey to find out if motivation sources might be linked to different types of discrimination. Express your conclusion either in graphical form or as a statistical analysis. Use a computer, save on disk, and print.

N2.1, 2.2, 2.3

IT2.1, 2.2, 2.3

2 You will find that the answers are not straightforward. Discuss why this should be so.

	X or ✔
talent	
pride	
upbringing	
religion	
role models	
money	
anger	
fear of failure	
encouragement	
the will to succeed	
health and energy	
ambition	
self-esteem	
other people's failure	

Maintaining confidentiality of information

Confidentiality is of critical importance in health and social care settings. It has a key role to play in client rights, client choices, and building trust. It is important to realise that there can be no such thing as **absolute confidentiality**; this is discussed on page 66.

NOTE BOOK
Advocacy is explained on page 75.

Client rights

Clients have equal rights with all citizens, which includes their rights to **privacy**, their own idea of **sexuality**, and **personal beliefs**.

They have a right to **information** about legal matters, grievance and complaints systems, and the need for their consent to certain treatments and procedures. This may involve the appointment of an **advocate**. Formal care settings have established procedures to protect rights which need to be understood equally by carers and their clients.

Client choices

Clients may need to be encouraged to say what they would prefer. Those who would be confused by too many options may need to be offered **guided choice**. This means that the choice is made less confusing by someone else first choosing a small number of equally suitable options. It is important that all workers in the establishment understand this and that it is explained to the client in a way that can be understood.

Choice includes matters of

- food
- clothing
- leisure activities
- independence.

Sometimes clients may make unwise choices which could put them or others at risk, or which would interfere with other people's rights. If this occurs it must be explained in a way that can be understood by those concerned. In the same way, clients' rights to choices have to be observed against the background of the care setting. Sometimes this limits the amount of choice available to clients.

Building trust

Often the carers delivering the most intimate care for clients, such as toileting and bathing, are those who may be regarded as being in the lowliest areas of work. These include care assistants, classroom assistants, and health care workers. Yet they are in a privileged position, as they receive many of the most personal and private confidences of clients. A close relationship is thus built, with the client placing great trust in the carer. Carers in administrative or senior positions may have moved away from this special friendship, and they

unit one

may rely on junior staff to discover aspects of clients' lives and personalities that are not directly concerned with treatment and care.

Clients need to know that their carers will treat any information they are given as confidential. In order to do this

- records containing clients' details are kept securely, according to the establishment's procedures

- written records should not contain explicit or unnecessary detail

- confidential information should be passed on in a suitably private environment

- anything of a personal nature relating to clients is never discussed outside the workplace.

The ethical issues that individuals may face in relation to maintaining confidentiality

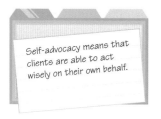

Self-advocacy means that clients are able to act wisely on their own behalf.

A further complexity in the relationship between client and carer is that of the **ethical nature** of the work. The health and social care services have a commitment to personal care and **self-advocacy**. They have deeply rooted ethical values to consider, if clients are not to be placed at a disadvantage, exploited, or damaged during the caring process.

It is difficult for any carer to promise full confidentiality to a client.

Here we will be examining over-riding confidentiality, disclosing information, and the balance between client rights and those of others.

Over-riding confidentiality

Carers have a dilemma if they learn something about a client which they think should be told to senior staff, while feeling a loyalty to the person in their care. The following reference points may help to clarify the situation.

1 Clients must be told in a way they can understand that sometimes personal information must be shared.

2 Such information is only given to those who need and have a right to know about it.

3 If confidential information reveals that anyone will be put at risk, it must be passed on. This could include

- information about drugs/medication being taken without the care team's knowledge

- information that the client plans to damage his or her own or other people's health or well-being

- personal information about past or present behaviour which may affect the client's treatment.

Disclosing information

Usually friends and family are involved when a client needs care. This widens the range of responsibility for carers who have to consider their professional duty to

- management

- colleagues

- clients

- clients' friends and families

- the public.

There may be times when a client is being coerced by those outside the care team to give information about treatment, domestic details, or maybe legal matters.

The same may happen to the carer, and it may be hard to decide how much or how little information to share. The following table lists some important principles about disclosing information.

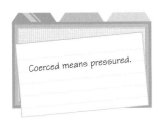

Coerced means pressured.

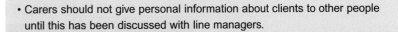

- Carers should not give personal information about clients to other people until this has been discussed with line managers.

- Clients should be protected by their carers against stressful pressure from others. Again, guidance should be sought from senior staff.

- Carers should not agree to act as witnesses for clients or their relatives or friends unless this has been expressly approved by senior management, and certainly never if they are below the age of 18.

Promoting and supporting individuals' rights to dignity, independence, health and safety

The balance between clients' rights and the rights of others

A client's well-being has always to be considered within the context of the organisation providing care. This means that everybody else has to be thought of at the same time:

- other clients

- their family and friends

- care staff
- others connected with the partcular client's care plan.

All clients have a right to **privacy** and dignity, whatever their age and level of understanding, and whether or not they are conscious.

Privacy means that you

- prevent other people from prying into clients' business
- discuss personal details in a way that cannot be overheard
- make sure that clothes are arranged modestly and avoid exposing the body more than you can help when giving intimate care to clients.

Dignity means that you

- always treat clients as individuals
- protect them from ridicule if their behaviour is unusual
- maintain a sympathetic and reassuring attitude at all times
- clean them up as best you can if they are sick or soil themselves
- ensure that your manner and speech are always courteous, kindly, and professional.

ACTIVITY C

C2.1a, 2.3 Discuss and record possible conflict of rights in the situations below.

- In residential care, other people's routines may dictate that eccentric time-keeping has to be discouraged.
- Loud music is thought inconsiderate when it disturbs others.
- Pregnant women may prefer not to have a male midwife.
- An able-bodied caving society feels unable to cater for the needs of a visually impaired student who wants to participate.
- An Asian woman speaking very little English applies to work in a residential setting with English-speaking young people with communication difficulties.

Independence

The balance in this aspect of our lifestyles is especially delicate, as all independence carries a degree of risk. Some carers use this as an excuse to pamper and mollycoddle clients, which some of them enjoy, but which is disempowering as it means that the carer is in charge of another person's life. It is also physically as well as emotionally damaging, as the body that doesn't move about deteriorates.

A person who is independent is one who is able to be free from the control of others. This may involve physical, emotional, or financial support from carers or the community.

Health and safety

Carers need to be aware of risks to health and safety in the immediate surroundings – both inside and out – to help them learn how to reduce the likelihood of accidents. We are constantly surrounded by danger. Safety is to do with recognising dangers, or **hazards**, and keeping the risks they pose under control. Those who need looking after may not be able to recognise these hazards. So we must be on the alert to make sure that their surroundings are made as safe as possible without placing too many restrictions on individuals' independence.

The secret of reducing the risk of accidents is to use everything for its intended purpose, and to keep surroundings tidy. Muddle creates muddle and encourages muddled thinking. Fewer accidents happen in a tidy and controlled environment.

It is a sad fact that most accidents occur in people's own homes, so we need to look first at safety right under our noses – in the home and garden, on the road, in social settings, and in the local environment.

Hazards in the home and garden

ACTIVITY D

Look at the table on the right and over the page, and then draw connecting lines linking the hazard with the risk. One is done for you as an example.

a KITCHEN	RISK	HAZARD
	Fire	Refrigerator
	Burns and scalds	Hot pans
	Cuts	Waste bin
	Infection	Cleaning materials
	Poisoning	Electrical equipment
	Tripping/falling	Knives
	Electrocution	Cooker
		Mats
		Spilt food

b BATHROOM	RISK	HAZARD
	Scalding	Electrical equipment
	Poisoning	Bath
	Falling	Shampoo
	Cuts	Water
	Drowning	Lavatory
	Infection	Tablets
	Allergies	Flannels
	Electrocution	Bath mats
		Soap/bubble bath
		Taps

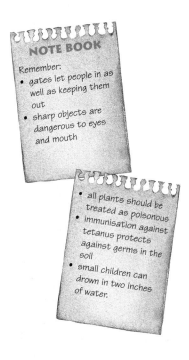

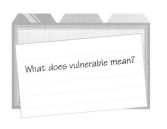

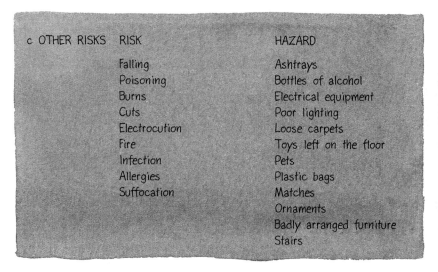

c OTHER RISKS RISK	HAZARD
Falling	Ashtrays
Poisoning	Bottles of alcohol
Burns	Electrical equipment
Cuts	Poor lighting
Electrocution	Loose carpets
Fire	Toys left on the floor
Infection	Pets
Allergies	Plastic bags
Suffocation	Matches
	Ornaments
	Badly arranged furniture
	Stairs

ACTIVITY E

Opposite is a plan of a garden. Make a list of the places in this garden where you think there could be possible health hazards.

What does vulnerable mean?

Poisonous plants

Small children, and older people who are confused or have problems understanding the world around them, tend to put things into their mouths, either to explore them out of curiosity, or because they are hungry. Unpleasant tastes, curiously enough, do not discourage them. Berries are tempting and attractive, but all parts of a plant should be regarded as poisonous – flowers, leaves, seeds, and berries. It is a good idea to avoid growing plants known to be poisonous where there are vulnerable people.

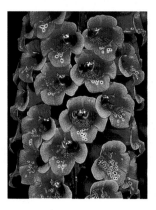
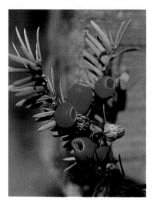
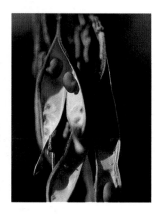
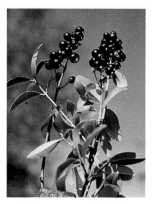

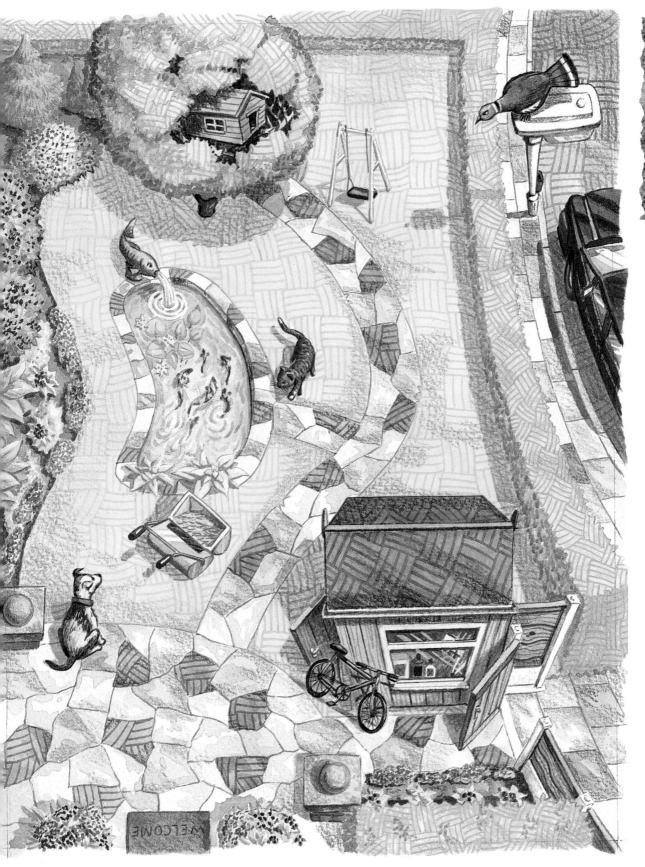

Acknowledging individuals' personal beliefs and identity

When communication between client and carer is effective, then something positive emerges. The positive aspects examined here are client empowerment, acknowledgement of personal beliefs and identity, building self-esteem, and building self-confidence.

Client empowerment

When someone is empowered, they are given strength, which means emotional strength rather than physical power. Here we will explore how a carer can give a client power of his or her own. Because of traditional views of patients and others who need looking after, clients often fall into an expected role of dependence, and it can be quite difficult to 'give them permission' to exercise power of their own.

It is achieved by

- letting them know this is acceptable
- encouraging independence
- giving access to choices
- education in life skills as well as traditional subjects
- maximising communication skills
- getting to know clients as individuals and allowing them to be themselves
- helping them to behave as accepted members of society.

Acknowledgement of personal beliefs and identity

Before clients can develop their own beliefs they need access to ideas and concepts, and help in understanding them.

With many this takes place during their childhood, and their beliefs may be firmly established before they are in need of care. For those who are 'clients' from infancy, or who may be brought up in institutions, it is part of the caring role to provide opportunities for spiritual enrichment and discussion of abstract opinions within the client's abilities. In this way people discover who they are.

If individuals are given stereotyping labels their identity is lost and they cease to be seen as themselves. It works both ways – that is, both client and carer are often stereotyped. No one likes to be perceived merely as a role.

Carer and client need to see one another as individuals and accept each other's beliefs, whether or not they are shared.

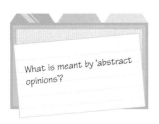

What is meant by 'abstract opinions'?

Building self-confidence

Empowerment + a feeling of identity + high self-esteem = self-confidence. This literally means being confident in one's self rather than relying on others. The media tell of many individuals who we might expect to be overwhelmingly handicapped by illness, misfortune, or disability, who nevertheless run in marathons, write books, achieve awards, and pursue fulfilling careers against all the odds.

This shows that with certain advantages everyone can grow into a self-reliant person, capable of operating independently within their abilities. They sometimes achieve beyond anyone's expectations.

The factors contributing to the self-confidence of individuals are

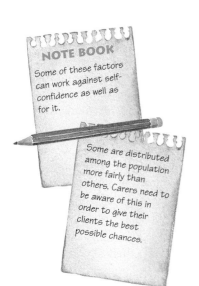

NOTE BOOK
Some of these factors can work against self-confidence as well as for it.

Some are distributed among the population more fairly than others. Carers need to be aware of this in order to give their clients the best possible chances.

- personality
- family
- quality of care
- dedication of carers
- support from the state
- effective treatment
- equality of access
- funds
- locality.

Supporting individuals through alternative approaches

Sometimes it is hard to find an appropriate way to help clients. We have already looked at the need for effective communication, which might need enhancing with hearing aids or communication boards. Another way of helping is to give clear information about services and how to access them, about rights within services, and the use of translators and advocates. A service is of little use if no one knows anything about it.

Services and how to access them

Information can be provided in a variety of ways:

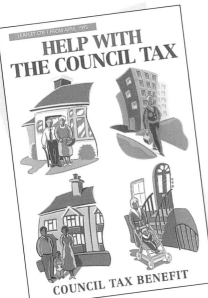

LEAFLET CTB 1 FROM APRIL 1995
HELP WITH
THE COUNCIL TAX

COUNCIL TAX BENEFIT

- paper-based – books

    – posters

    – leaflets, etc.
- on audiotapes
- on radio

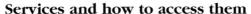

- on video or television
- word of mouth – formally, in schools, colleges, or lectures
  – informally, from friends and family.

The method of presentation is vitally important, and must be appropriate for the target group.

Here is a list of examples where appropriateness is important.

- A small percentage of elderly people in the UK are HIV-positive. Information on support and how to access it must be presented differently from that targeting young gay people.

- Young people in mainstream education need information on where they can have access to counselling. So do young people in a nearby school for students with moderate learning disabilities. The information needs presenting differently for each group.

- Visually impaired women have right of access to well-women clinics. It would not be appropriate to give this information visually in the same way as publicity aimed at sighted women.

- Individuals who do not use English as a first language need information in their own language and dialect. They also need access to health and social care workers who understand their culture and can pass on information sympathetically and realistically.

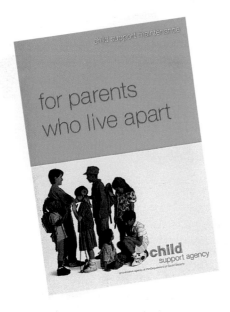

ACTIVITY F

1 List the places where you have seen information displayed on health and social care services.
2 What form did it take?
3 Do you think it was accessible to most of the public?
4 Do you think it would appeal to most of the public?
5 Was it understandable to those who would see it?
6 Record your information, mentioning percentages and ratios where you consider it appropriate.

N2.2

Information about rights within services

All clients have a right to

- **access to services**
- **confidentiality** – no information gained about them in the course of services being delivered must be shared outside the professional setting

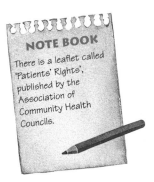

NOTE BOOK

There is a leaflet called 'Patients' Rights', published by the Association of Community Health Councils.

- **non-discriminatory treatment** – in the United Kingdom all clients are entitled to equal treatment, access to services, and quality of care. This is stated in all written policies connected with the health and social care services, the Patient's Charter, and the Community Care Charter. This means that no one should be discriminated against because they are of a different race or culture, or have different beliefs from the majority of the population. Males and females should be treated equally. People with disabilities should be on an equal footing with able-bodied people. An individual's age should not be held against them. In short, everyone should be treated in the same way.

Use of a translator

All clients have the right to be understood and to understand. This includes individuals who

- do not speak or understand English fluently

- are deaf and communicate through British Sign Language or in other ways

- have physical or learning disabilities which prevent them from understanding or speaking easily.

Where a client uses a service in a neighbourhood where their own language is not commonly used, they are entitled to the help of a translator if necessary. Others with communication problems are also entitled to help from someone used to their own way of 'speaking'.

Use of an advocate

An advocate is someone who responds on behalf of another person who is unable to act for him or herself. This is different from the service given by a translator, who only re-expresses what a person has actually said. Some areas have set up Citizen Advocacy Systems, working especially in the area of mental health and with clients who are disadvantaged or have learning difficulties. There are plans to extend this into a National Advocacy Network.

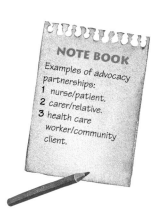

NOTE BOOK

Examples of advocacy partnerships:
1 nurse/patient.
2 carer/relative.
3 health care worker/community client.

Advocacy is about
- Helping people to speak up for themselves or speaking on their behalf if necessary
- Helping people to become involved in their own care and to become as independent as possible. This is called **self-advocacy** and **empowers** people.
- Ensuring that rights and choices are respected, and helping those who are disadvantaged or who have disabilities to participate as fully as possible in society.
- Making sure that the client has equal power with the service providers.
- Forming partnerships between client and advocate so that one can speak for the other in an impartial way in an atmosphere of trust and confidence.

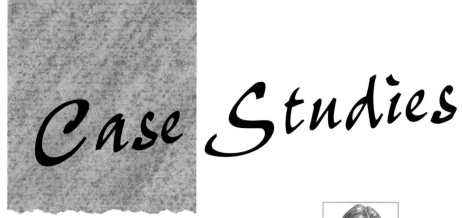

Case Studies

Case study 4.1   Down Way School
(continued from Unit 1.3)

Jalwinder goes out into the corridor to see if she can help and the father calls her 'a scrawny little Paki'. Jalwinder loses her temper, which is rare for her, and shouts back that the parent is discriminating against her. Later in the playground she overhears the children repeating 'scrawny little Paki' as the chorus to a skipping game.

Task 1

1   How could the staff at the school explain the meaning of discrimination to the children?

2   Would children find it easier to understand the short- or the long-term effects of discrimination?

Task 2

1   What forms of discrimination are being exhibited?

2   How is the discrimination being demonstrated?

Task 2

3   Is Gertrude being discriminatory, stereotyping, or neither?

4   Discuss your answers in a group.

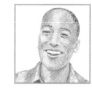

Case study 4.2   The Thatched Cottage

Mark takes some of the residents to the nearby pub every Thursday for a drink before lunch, pushing Bill in his wheelchair. He began the habit to celebrate his 18th birthday and has continued with it ever since. He gets annoyed with one of the bar staff who speaks to him instead of Bill when the drinks are being ordered, and with a woman who complains loudly about the residents lowering the tone of the establishment. Luckily the pub manager is on Mark's side, and has a word with the bar person, and makes it clear to the woman that The Thatched Cottage residents are always welcome. Gertrude finds this encouraging, and, after downing a glass of stout, launches into a graphic account of the joys of being bathed by Mark.

Case study 4.3   Hill Hall

Outside the walls of Hill Hall there is much opportunity for discrimination. Molly's race and colour and the children's learning difficulties and sometimes bizarre ways make them easy targets for discriminatory behaviour. Molly likes to take some of the children to a local hypermarket to help them to see everyday life. One day she is jostled by a shopper who tells her to get her 'great dirty hands off the bread'. One of the children catches Molly's distress and begins to throw buns at the shopper. The manager is called, and threatens the shopper with legal action. The shopper retaliates with a threat because there are no toilet adaptations for disabled people (which is irrelevant, but true).

Task 3

1   Which Acts could the manager and the shopper be penalised under?

2   If the hypermarket manager sacked a staff member because she was pregnant, or paid paperboys more than papergirls, which other Acts would be broken?

Case study 4.4   Netherfield Community Care

There is a significant degree of unemployment in the town. The prison service has a helpline for ex-offenders, and anyone needing a sympathetic ear can ring at any time of day or night. It becomes obvious that, after coming out of prison, the young men in particular are not being offered job interviews. The local community decides to address this matter.

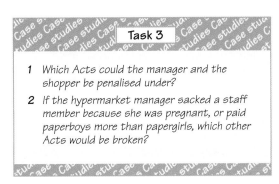

Task 4

1   What legislation is there in your area to help this group of people to secure jobs?

2   What are the likely effects of this sort of discrimination on the young men of Netherfield, which makes it desirable to act on their behalf before too much time passes?

Task 4

3   What might be the stereotyping which leads to discrimination against ex-offenders applying for jobs?

◀▶ Extension opportunity

Look in the media for evidence of discrimination leading to detrimental job prospects. Use the seven different forms of discrimination. Remember that 'the media' includes television, radio, and written material. Select an appropriate format for your findings. Employ Key Skills imaginatively.

Case study 4.5   Netherfield Community Care

It has been a bad day at the Community Care office. One of the clients with clinical depression has tried to commit suicide, and the team is having a meeting to discuss future management of her case. Debbie is included, as she had reported to Mikhail the week before that this client had told her in confidence that she intended to take her own life. The client had become distressed when Debbie had stated that she would have to report the information, and Debbie feels guilty that she may have contributed to the client's action.

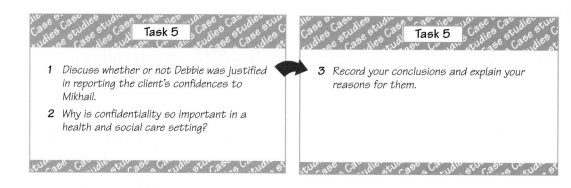

Task 5

1 Discuss whether or not Debbie was justified in reporting the client's confidences to Mikhail.

2 Why is confidentiality so important in a health and social care setting?

Task 5

3 Record your conclusions and explain your reasons for them.

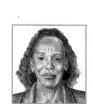

Case study 4.6   Hill Hall

Ann is impressed by Molly's professionalism. She always seems to know exactly how to respond, even in unexpected circumstances. One day a relative of one of the children asks very persistently for information about treatment and the child's possible progress. Molly is very cool and business-like in her response. When they discuss this over coffee one day, Molly is a bit off-hand, and says 'It's dead easy; you just have to think of them all as special people, and realise at the same time that we all have to get on together here.' Ann mentions this in class when she gets back to college, and they discuss the ethical issues involved.

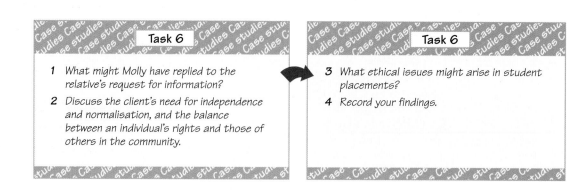

Task 6

1 What might Molly have replied to the relative's request for information?

2 Discuss the client's need for independence and normalisation, and the balance between an individual's rights and those of others in the community.

Task 6

3 What ethical issues might arise in student placements?

4 Record your findings.

Multiple Choice Questions

4.1 Calling someone a 'white fascist' is an example of discriminatory behaviour which is

   a *covert*

   b *indirect*

   c *overt*

   d *sexist*

4.2 Which of the following is an example of a basis for discrimination?

   a *anger*

   b *age*

   c *motivation*

   d *stereotype*

4.3 Which of the following might be a long-term effect of discrimination?

   a *lack of motivation*

   b *abusive language*

   c *stereotyping*

   d *indirect behaviour*

4.4 Which action would best be described as *indirect* discriminatory behaviour?

   a *touching someone believed to be HIV-positive*

   b *using abusive language to a confused client*

   c *ignoring a person in a wheelchair*

   d *using a tone of voice which ridicules a Chinese woman*

4.5 Stereotyping means

   a *thinking that all people in a group are the same*

   b *behaving badly towards people with disabilities*

   c *avoiding people who have a different religion*

   d *telling racist jokes*

4.6 Which of the following Acts makes it compulsory for architects to design public buildings with ramps for access?

   a *the Race Relations Act*

   b *the Sex Discrimination Act*

   c *the Equal Pay Act*

   d *the Disabled Persons Act*

4.7 Balancing clients' rights with those of others is an issue of

   a *ethnics*

   b *confidentiality*

   c *ethics*

   d *acknowledgement*

4.8 Which statement best describes the importance of confidentiality?

   a *it respects clients' rights and builds trust*

   b *it gives clients physical support in the community*

   c *it is one of the differences between formal and informal care*

   d *it is part of the dependence of clients*

Multiple Choice Questions

4.9 Effective interaction in caring means

a providing support for clients

b helping clients to become dependent

c undertaking daily living tasks for clients

d empowering the client

4.10 Which of the following is a valid reason for over-riding confidentiality?

a when the client responds aggressively

b acknowledge the client's identity

c when the caring relationship is at risk

d when the carer is uncertain of his/her ability to respond effectively

Note: These questions are for you to test your knowledge. There is no formal multiple choice test in this GNVQ.

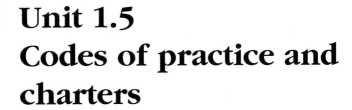

Unit 1.5
Codes of practice and charters

The care value base is used in the production of documents supporting clients' rights. These help to protect clients and give them an effective route for expressing their views, opinions, and complaints.

Examples of such documents, incorporating many features of the care value base, include the code of practice used in residential care and the Patient's Charter. They can be seen in libraries or obtained from relevant organisations. The Patient's Charter is often displayed in doctors' surgeries.

If you take part in out-of-school/college work activities, it is likely that the care and child care organisations in which you gain your work experience have copies of their own particular codes of practice and charters.

ACTIVITY A

Find details of as many different codes of practice and charters as you can, by looking in your library, using HMSO (Her Majesty's Stationery Office) or government websites, or contacting your local authority or local social services enquiry departments.

File the information you collect with your main Unit 1 assessment.

| C2.2 | IT2.1, 2.2, 2.3 |

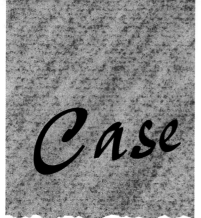

Case Study

**Case study 5.1   Netherfield Community Care, Hill Hall,
                    The Thatched Cottage, and Down Way School**

Debbie, Ann, Mark, and Jalwinder have been discussing the
similarities and differences between their four work places in
their application of the care value base. Not all of them can
remember seeing any code of practice or anything like a patients'
charter on display.

Task 1

1   Working as a group, combine your findings
    from Activity A (page 81). Decide which
    codes of practice and charters might be
    used by the Netherfield Community Care
    team, at Hill Hall and Down Way schools,
    and at The Thatched Cottage.

Task 1

2   Relate the contents to the care value base
    and the support of client rights.

Compulsory Assessment Activity

Evidence for Unit One

Here is an outline of the main evidence you are required to produce in order to be successful in Unit One. The optional tasks and activities described throughout the unit chapter (pages 15-82) have been designed to make it easier for you to complete this final compulsory piece of work. Your teaching staff need to approve your chosen topic, so the following information intentionally gives only broad guidance.

You must produce a report based on two different health and/or social care settings, including

- a description of the way the services are organised, and the roles of the people who work with them

- an explanation of the care value base that underpins all work in supporting clients in both settings

- an exploration of the importance and application of communication skills in care settings.

In order to achieve a pass, you must show that you can understand and use relevant information to

- correctly identify the care sector and client group of both your chosen settings (see page 16, *The organisation of health, social care, and early years services*)

- clearly describe the roles of two workers, correctly identifying and explaining the care value base that would underpin their work (see page 23, *The main jobs in health, social care, and early years services*, and page 55, *The care value base*)

- describe the use of any codes of practice or charters that relate to the organisation in which the workers are based (see page 81, *Codes of practice and charters*)

- demonstrate relevant communication skills (see page 37, *Effective communication skills*)

- describe possible barriers to communication with clients (see page 37, *Effective communication skills*).

If you are keen to gain a merit or distinction, your work will need to be more complex. Your teacher or lecturer will tell you how to achieve these higher grades.

Summary of evidence opportunities

1.1 The organisation of health, social care, and early years services

Activities A (page 18), B (page 18), C (page 19), D (page 19)

Case studies 1.1, 1.2, 1.3, 1.4 (pages 20-21)

1.2 Main jobs in health, social care, and early years services

Activity A (page 29)

Case studies 2.1, 2.2, 2.3, 2.4 (pages 34-35)

1.3 Effective communication skills

Activities A (page 38), B (page 42), C (page 45), D (page 46), E (page 46), F (page 47), G (page 48), H (page 49), I (page 50), J (page 51), K (page 51)

Case studies 3.1, 3.2, 3.3, 3.4 (pages 52-53)

1.4 The care value base

Activities A (page 62), B (page 64), C (page 68), D (page 69), E (page 70), F (page 74)

Case studies 4.1, 4.2, 4.3, 4.4, 4.5, 4.6 (pages 76-78)

1.5 Codes of practice and charters

Activity A (page 81)

Case study 5.1 (page 82)

Personal evidence tracking record

Remember that you can use portfolio evidence more than once, to show understanding of other units.

unit one

1.1 The organisation of health, social care, and early years services	Description of evidence	Portfolio reference number
Statutory sector organisations		
NHS		
local authority services		
Voluntary organisations		
Private organisations		
Informal care		

1.2 Main jobs in health, social care, and early years services		
Direct care		
Indirect care		

1.3 Effective communication skills		
Listening and responding		
Non-verbal communication		
Questioning		
Appropriate use of language		

1.4 The care value base		
Anti-discriminatory practice		
Confidentiality		
Individuals' rights		
Individuals' personal beliefs and identity		
Alternative approaches		

1.5 Codes of practice and charters		
Codes of practice		
Charters		

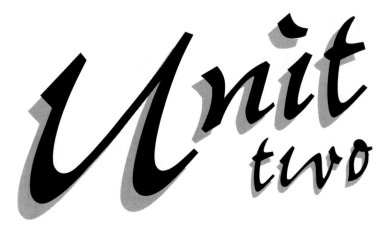

Promoting Health and Well-being

Introduction

In this unit you will learn

- definitions of health and well-being
- aspects of health and well-being that differ between different people and groups of people
- common factors that affect health and well-being and the different effects they can have on people
- physical measures that can be used to estimate health.

This unit is assessed through your portfolio work, and the grade you are given will be your grade for the unit.

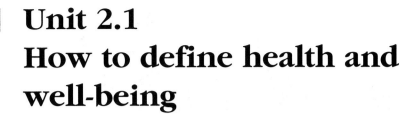

Unit 2.1
How to define health and well-being

Having a feeling of health and well-being means enjoying 'positive health' – and this means more than 'good health', which could be taken to mean just the absence of ill health. Positive health is possible for everyone, whatever their age, even when they have a persistent or incurable illness, have problems understanding things, or have a physical disability.

In your work you may need to give careful advice to your clients, as they could have difficulty understanding how to reach a balance in their lives. If all goes well, they will achieve a state of well-being. It is to do with accepting who we are, managing our lives effectively, and selecting a lifestyle that will help us to develop positive health.

You will learn the ways in which the health of individuals can be improved, regardless of age, ability, or way of life. You will also learn how to encourage your clients to follow a healthy lifestyle so that their health can be maintained and they do not harm themselves by doing things that might damage their bodies or minds.

unit two

The importance of a balanced lifestyle

Our bodies and minds are designed to work as a whole; one affects the other. Health care which takes the whole person into account, rather than just treating one part, is called 'holistic' – which comes from the theory of 'holism'.

We are constantly changing due to the influence of our own internal body systems – for example, our hormones, our response to illness, and ageing. We are also influenced by things outside ourselves – for example, the behaviour of other people, demands of work, and accidents. Whether the changes are enjoyable or unpleasant, they all mean that our bodies and minds have to be constantly adjusting in order to maintain a balance in our lives.

Ideally, lifestyles are balanced in terms of

> **activity** – work and recreation
>
> **rest** – sleep and inactivity.

Look at the see-saw diagram at the top of the next page. It shows factors affecting the balance of good health. Neither side is better than the other. The important thing is that the factors affecting lifestyle should be balanced effectively for each individual.

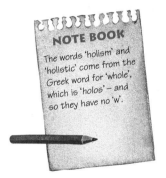

NOTE BOOK

The words 'holism' and 'holistic' come from the Greek word for 'whole', which is 'holos' – and so they have no 'w'.

Factors affecting the balance of good health

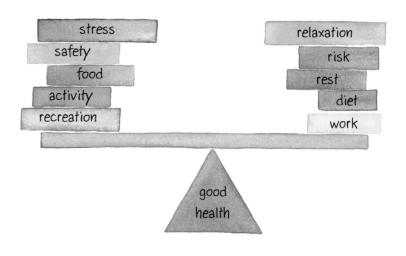

ACTIVITY A

Make a diagram illustrating the see-saw of your own lifestyle, using the same factors as those in the diagram above. Do it in rough, so you can make the sides go up and down if you think the importance of one activity is weightier than another. You will make a final copy later on.

Our physical needs are similar to those of the rest of the animal kingdom. Like them, we need to be safe and comfortable, with adequate supplies of air, water, food, shelter, and warmth; enough rest, sleep, and activity; and opportunities for sexual expression. Intellectual and spiritual refreshment, creativity, personal satisfaction, self-esteem, and feelings of achievement, like the need for love and approval, are more complicated needs for well-being. All needs vary between individuals and at different ages in life.

A person with disabilities has the same needs for healthy living, and for independence, as any other member of society. (See Unit One, page 23.)

In the 1950s, a psychologist called Abraham Maslow produced a definition of all individuals' needs, whatever their gender, age, or level of personal health. Maslow's 'Hierarchy of Needs' is shown opposite. Together, the needs he identified are a summary of all the physical, social, intellectual, and emotional needs for health and well-being.

The needs listed as 1, 2, and 3 allow for physical growth. The needs listed as 3, 4, and 5 allow for personal growth. You will notice that the need for love and belonging appears in both categories.

The benefits from needs 3, 4, and 5 can only be achieved when the needs from 1 and 2 have been satisfied. For example, it is almost impossible to concentrate on fulfilling one's potential when one is cold and hungry.

What is an individual?

A dictionary definition of the word 'individual' is 'single, having distinct character'. When we talk about people as being individuals, we acknowledge that there is something special and distinctive about each one of them.

Individuals in society are of all ages – babies, children, adolescents, adults, those in mid-life, and older people. They will all have their own personalities – kind, grumpy, quiet, boisterous, dramatic, etc. They may be pregnant. They may be in good health or be ill, be very academic or rather practical, physically fit or physically disabled. Their way of life may be active or sedentary (which means sitting down), exciting or boring, rewarding or demanding.

All of them will be a mixture of age, personality, health status, and way of life and will need to be respected accordingly by those whom they meet. You too are an individual and have your own needs.

The way of life that each individual chooses has a great impact on their health and well-being. Their chosen lifestyle, along with cultural influences, affects their health and well-being needs. Certain living and working conditions impose severe restrictions on an individual's ability to choose a healthy lifestyle.

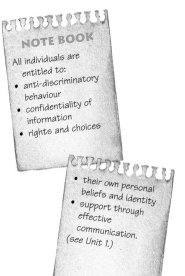

NOTE BOOK

All individuals are entitled to:
- anti-discriminatory behaviour
- confidentiality of information
- rights and choices

- their own personal beliefs and identity
- support through effective communication.
(see Unit 1.)

unit two

Maslow's Hierarchy of Needs

1. Need for survival
food, drink, shelter, sleep, etc – all physical needs

2. Need for safety
a stable and predictable environment, free from physical, psychological, or economic anxiety

3. Need for love and belonging
affection and intimacy from partners, family, and group

4. Need for esteem
self-confidence, recognition, appreciation, and respect from others

5. Need for self-actualisation
discovering and fulfilling one's own potential

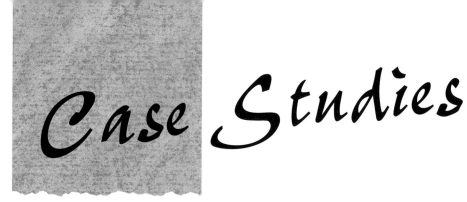

Case Studies

The students at The Thatched Cottage, with the health care team in Netherfield, and at Down Way School all have to prepare case studies in which they work out the different needs of their clients.

Case study 1.1 The Thatched Cottage

Rosa is a resident with age-related confusion. She is an identical twin, and became deaf in one ear when she was a child. She lives with her husband in a twin room in The Thatched Cottage, having moved from a large rambling house to be nearer her family. Mark is preparing a case study to identify Rosa's specific needs.

As a child, Rosa was isolated by her deafness. Her twin sister has remained a source of strength all her life. To them both, their religious faith has been a focal point for their friendships; their father was a parson. Rosa's husband enjoys listening to music, but Rosa, of course, cannot share his pleasure; she used to enjoy reading and writing poetry before she became too confused.

Case study 1.2 Netherfield Community Care

Debbie becomes interested in Mishka, a widow from Poland living in the town. She speaks little English, but can understand it quite well. Her son was diagnosed as having schizophrenia, and Mishka was devastated when he began to live rough, although things have improved since he came under the care of the health care team. Debbie asks Mikhail to help her to ask Mishka if she can use her experiences for a case study in which she will identify Mishka's needs for health and well-being.

Mishka has developed a friendship with the eccentric caretaker of her block of flats. Debbie cannot understand why they get on – Mishka is proudly Polish, the man is English. Mishka is rather aristocratic and reserved, while the caretaker is, quite frankly, rather scruffy and outward-going. He accepts Mishka's son's illness calmly, and lets him sleep in the boiler-room when the weather is poor.

Case study 1.3 Down Way School

Jalwinder would like to prepare a case study about Tim. He came to the school very withdrawn and apparently able to speak only a few words. Six months later he is chatty and settling well. He lives down the road from Jalwinder, and Isabel knows his mother well.

Jalwinder and Tim are getting to know one another well. She helps him to cut up his lunch and ties his shoe laces. When there is a dispute in the playground, he runs to her for support, as he is frightened of being bullied. Isabel recommends to Jalwinder that she should encourage Tim to be more independent. He has an imaginary friend who lives at the bottom of the garden and never comes into the house until it is dark. His mother has been asking Isabel if she 'ought to do something' about the friend, as Tim talks to 'it' at night and it is getting on her nerves.

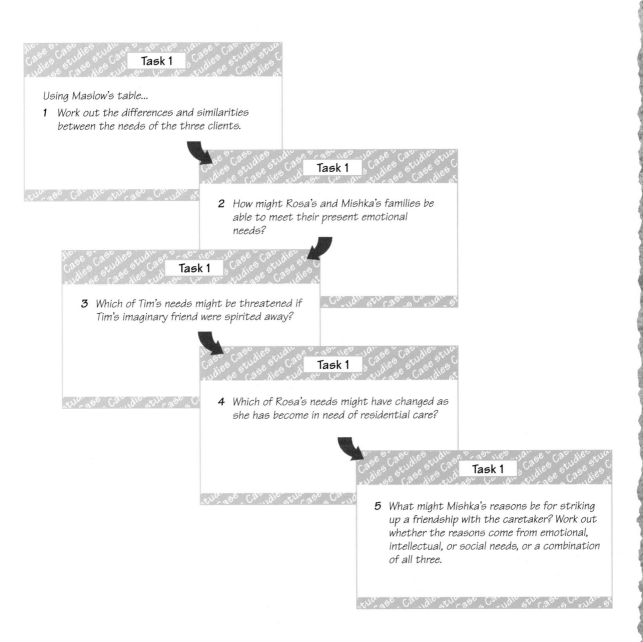

Task 1

Using Maslow's table...

1   Work out the differences and similarities between the needs of the three clients.

Task 1

2   How might Rosa's and Mishka's families be able to meet their present emotional needs?

Task 1

3   Which of Tim's needs might be threatened if Tim's imaginary friend were spirited away?

Task 1

4   Which of Rosa's needs might have changed as she has become in need of residential care?

Task 1

5   What might Mishka's reasons be for striking up a friendship with the caretaker? Work out whether the reasons come from emotional, intellectual, or social needs, or a combination of all three.

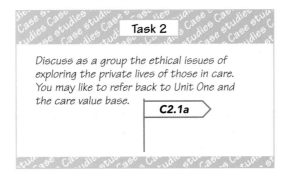

Task 2

Discuss as a group the ethical issues of exploring the private lives of those in care. You may like to refer back to Unit One and the care value base.

C2.1a

unit two **case studies**

Multiple Choice Questions

1.1 Positive health means

   a *health care is given by the National Health Service*

   b *enjoying good health and well-being*

   c *diabetics receive regular medication*

   d *a society has a clean water supply*

1.2 A balanced lifestyle is one which

   a *benefits both mind and body*

   b *allows individuals to do what they want*

   c *gives adequate work and activity*

   d *has a balanced diet*

1.3 Which of the following is most likely to have a lifestyle that might not support health and well-being needs?

   a *a new baby*

   b *a New Age traveller*

   c *a homeless adolescent*

   d *an elderly widow*

1.4 Which of the following is important for physical growth?

   a *adequate sleep*

   b *respect from others*

   c *discovering one's potential*

   d *self-actualisation*

Note: These questions are for you to test your knowledge. There is no formal multiple choice test in this GNVQ.

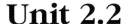

Unit 2.2
Factors affecting health and well-being

There are many factors affecting a person's health and well-being. They include diet, exercise, and social factors such as environment, social class, employment, housing, income, and education. These all combine to have different effects on each individual's physical, emotional, social, and intellectual health, and on their well-being.

People can put themselves at risk because of what they choose to do or what they choose not to do. Increased health risks are the result of substance abuse (including legal and illegal drugs, alcohol, and tobacco), poor diet, stress, poor personal hygiene, lack of physical exercise, unsafe sexual behaviour, or dangerous workplace activities. These topics are covered together in the following section.

Risks and benefits associated with aspects of lifestyles

Any lifestyle which excludes any of the needs listed below might place the individual's health at risk.

Needs for positive health

1 Exercise – benefits the body by

- improving muscle tone
- keeping the blood and lymphatic circulation moving
- increasing lung capacity
- keeping joints mobile
- helping digestion
- preventing constipation
- promoting well-being and reducing depression.

Exercise needs to be balanced with rest. An active child needs to have periods of quiet during which active muscles can recover. A person in a wheelchair needs to do regular exercises to counteract long hours sitting still.

Fitness and exercise are not concerned with the number of press-ups people can do or how far they can jog, but more with the strength and flexibility of their bodies. These are affected by an individual's

- state of health and presence of illness or disability

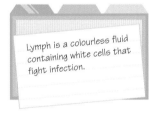

Lymph is a colourless fluid containing white cells that fight infection.

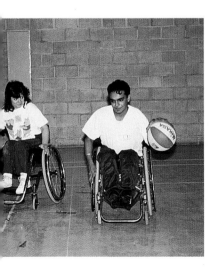

unit two

- age

- weight

- lung efficiency

- exercise levels and physical agility

- personality and attitude.

2 **A balanced diet** – contains nutrients in the right proportions to maintain body health.

3 **Sufficient rest and recreation** – allow the body and mind to recover after activity. In some cultures this is called 'allowing the soul to catch up'.

4 **Not smoking** – maintains the lungs in a clean condition and greatly reduces the possibility of bronchitis, lung cancer, and heart disease in the smoker and other people.

5 **Avoidance of alcohol abuse**. A sensible approach to drinking alcohol prevents dependency, liver and brain deterioration, and the possibility of breakdown of relationships. It is generally thought that small amounts of alcohol are not harmful to the body.

6 **Safe sexual behaviour, including celibacy**. A responsible attitude to sexual behaviour lessens the likelihood of contracting diseases such as AIDS, hepatitis B, genital warts, herpes, gonorrhea, and cervical cancer.

Safe sexual behaviour includes:

- paying attention to personal hygiene after sex

- not having many sexual partners

- using a condom. This applies to heterosexual and homosexual partners

- celibacy, which means not having sexual relationships at all.

Selecting an appropriate lifestyle

How balanced is your lifestyle?

Do you ever give yourself treats?
Is your working life satisfactory?
Does your work expand into your home life?*
Is your emotional life good?
How are your money matters?
Are you living where you want to?
Is your way of life healthy?

*Remember that 'work' includes study and voluntary work, as well as paid work.

Are your treats good for you?
Do you get what you want from your holidays?
Do you enjoy your leisure time?
Could you spend more time with the people you care about?
Are you claiming all your benefits?
Could you improve your living space?
Would you feel happier if you ate/drank/exercised differently?

ACTIVITY A

Return to the rough copy of your lifestyle which you made in Activity A of Unit 2.1 (page 88) and see if it needs adjusting. Make a good copy for your portfolio; it will provide evidence to demonstrate that you have thought about the importance of a balanced lifestyle.

The lifestyle chosen by individuals tells us much about their personality and philosophy of living. However, not everyone can choose where they work or live, and it can cause stress and dissatisfaction when there is conflict between the dream of how you would like to live and the reality of your situation.

How the body uses each dietary component

Food is principally made up of proteins, carbohydrates, fat, vitamins and minerals, water, and fibre. Most of us give little thought to these and concentrate on what we like or what is available. When you look after other people, however, you need to understand about the make-up of food, as you may be called upon to provide low-fat, low-salt, high-fibre, or other specialist diets.

Protein is what we are made of. It is the building material of our bodies. As our cells are constantly dying and being replaced – more quickly during some illnesses – protein is essential for us to flourish and grow and for damaged tissues to be repaired.

Carbohydrates provide the fuel for us to work. They are divided into starches and sugars. All carbohydrates have to be converted into glucose before they can be used by the body. This process takes longer for starches than sugars. This means that starches take longer than sugars to digest and are more useful than sugars in stopping people from becoming hungry. It was once thought that carbohydrates alone caused people to put on weight. However, they are now seen as a valuable part of our diet. Individuals who use a lot of energy need to eat more carbohydrates to replace the energy that has been burnt up.

Fats are provided from animal or vegetable sources. The ones that are associated with harming the body by increasing the cholesterol level mostly come from animals, and are known as **saturated fats**. In general, vegetable fats are less harmful to our bodies, and are mostly known as **unsaturated fats**.

Fats provide twice the energy of carbohydrates and help proteins to carry out growth and repair, so while a low-fat diet is a healthy one, the body could not function if fats were excluded altogether.

Vitamins and minerals. Minute amounts of vitamins and minerals are needed to help the work of the proteins, carbohydrates, and fats. Some minerals are important in themselves. Calcium builds up the structure of our bones and teeth. Iron maintains the health of our red blood cells. An ordinary balanced diet contains adequate vitamins and minerals. It is only when there are greater demands on the body, such as during pregnancy or illness, that the average daily amounts need to be supplemented.

Fresh food is the best source of vitamins, as they deteriorate during storage or careless cooking. Vitamin C is found in fresh fruit and vegetables. It is important for the health of our skin, and helps the healing process in the body.

Vitamin D comes from fatty foods like margarine, eggs, and fish containing fats. It is also made by our skin during exposure to sunlight. It is essential for healthy bones and teeth.

Water. If we were squeezed dry, more than half the volume of our bodies would be found to be made of water. Much of our body systems' energy is spent keeping the water, and the nutrients dissolved in it, in the right place. The balance is affected by our fluid intake and output, which changes with the body's temperature and that of the surroundings and the amount of exercise taken. So we perspire and need to drink more when we are hot or exercising, and pass more urine when we are cold or resting.

The general requirement for fluid intake is about 1–1.5 litres (2 to 3 pints) daily. We **gain fluids** from all that we drink and much that we eat, and **lose fluids** by breathing, sweating, and passing urine and, to a lesser extent, faeces.

Some substances increase the passing of urine. These are called **diuretics**. Caffeine is one and alcohol is another. Also there are several diuretic medicines prescribed for people with fluid retention problems. Remember that fat cells contain very little water, so diuretics alone do not help in weight reduction. The table below looks at factors affecting fluid loss.

Factors affecting fluid loss

+ = increased
− = decreased

Factor	Body's response		
	urine output	sweating	thirst
heat	−	+	+
cold	+	−	−
exercise	−	+	+
raised body temperature	−	+	+
diuretics	+	+	normal

Fibre. Fibre used to be called roughage, and was valued mainly in preventing constipation. Now it is also thought to give protection against diseases of the large intestine, and to help in lowering the amount of cholesterol in the blood.

A healthy diet for an individual

Eating patterns

Our eating habits are affected by subtle psychological influences. We learn them from our families, friends, and the society in which we live. We use food as a bribe, as a reward, as a treat, or to comfort ourselves, as much as to satisfy hunger. Healthy eating has as much to do with our acceptance of ourselves as we are as it has to do with knowing the nutrients included in meals. Our appetites are often controlled by our emotions rather than our body's needs. Good carers never forget this when advising people about food, diet, and feeding habits.

The following table lists good and bad habits which contribute to a healthy diet.

Eating habits

GOOD HABITS	BAD HABITS
• keeping food out of sight between meals • not cooking too much, allowing for reasonable portions only • sitting down to eat • keeping to proper mealtimes • using minimal salt in cooking • keeping junk food out of the house	• smothering food with salt and relishes • finishing leftovers • using food for reward, or love substitute • eating on the move • 'grazing' continuously • bingeing then fasting • too much junk food

unit two

Healthy eating around the world

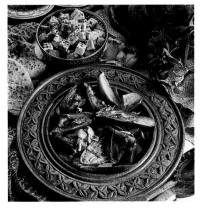

The Caribbean

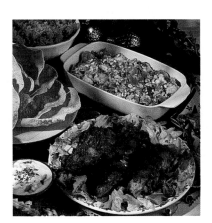

India

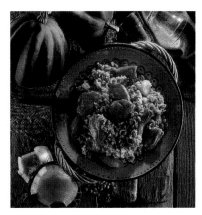

The Middle East

The types of food that should be eaten

- **proteins** such as meat, fish, dairy produce, pulses

- **carbohydrates** from starches such as potatoes, bread, and pasta rather than sugars

- not too much **fat**, especially saturated animal fat

- **vitamins**, **minerals**, and **fibre** from fresh fruit and vegetables

- **fibre** from whole foods, which tend to be 'brown' – e.g. brown rice, brown wholemeal bread, brown flour

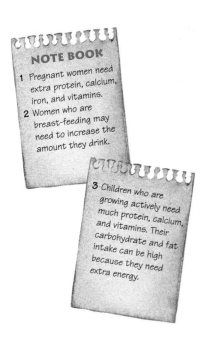

NOTE BOOK

1 Pregnant women need extra protein, calcium, iron, and vitamins.

2 Women who are breast-feeding may need to increase the amount they drink.

3 Children who are growing actively need much protein, calcium, and vitamins. Their carbohydrate and fat intake can be high because they need extra energy.

- not too much **salt** – do not add much during cooking, do not sprinkle it on after cooking

- not too much **sugar** or sweet food

- plenty of **fluids**, but not too much caffeine from tea or coffee (water is quite nice …)

- not too much **instant food and drink** – they contain additives and have lost much of their food value during preparation.

The right amount to eat

See Activity B.

ACTIVITY B

Extension opportunity

1 Find out the daily intake of food recommended by the following bodies:
   - NACNE – the National Advisory Committee on Nutrition Education
   - COMA – the Committee on Medical Aspects of Food Policy
   - JACNE – the Department of Health and the Joint Advisory Committee on Nutritional Education.

2 State how you found the information.

3 Record what you discover.
   Diet breakdown can be illustrated effectively using percentages, fractions, and decimal fractions. Use numerical information when you record this activity.

Recommended daily intake of foods for an adult (see also Department of Health recommended diet – pie chart page 114)

Protein
half pint/250ml of milk
1 egg
average serving of: cheese, fish, nuts, peas, beans, lentils, meat

Carbohydrate
starches – freely but not in excess
sugars – only enough to make food enjoyable

Fruits and vegetables
3 to 5 servings

Water
at least 1 pint/500ml

Fats
only enough to make food enjoyable
a animal fats • meat
• butter and some hard margarines
• full-fat dairy produce

b vegetable fats • sunflower oil
• vegetable margarine

c made-up foods • crisps
• cakes
• biscuits
• chocolate

The effects of use of substances on health and well-being

Any substance taken into the body will have an effect on it. The effect may be

- physical
- social
- emotional
- intellectual.

Substances may be natural or manufactured. We will be examining drugs intended for use in medical treatment, misuse of drugs intended for use in medical treatment, use of drugs which have no intended use in medical treatment, and misuse of solvents.

ACTIVITY C

Read through the following list of the possible effects of misusing substances:

- contracting diseases such as hepatitis B and AIDS which can be spread during intravenous injection of substances
- the break-up of relationships with friends and family
- difficulty in coping with a job
- dependency – which means being unable to manage without something

- exposure to the danger of taking to crime to pay for the habit
- destruction of brain cells
- change in mental state
- inability to exercise control over one's actions
- mood swings.

Decide whether these effects can be classed as physical, social, emotional, or intellectual .

Record your decision, to use when you come to the case studies on pages 108-109.

Drugs intended as medical treatment

Drug is another word for medicine. There are many thousands of drugs. Some commonly used ones are cough mixture, aspirin, and digoxin (a medicine given to regulate the heartbeat).

Many people are kept well by taking drugs regularly – think about those with diabetes or epilepsy. It is all to do with balance. The dose is regulated by the severity of the person's condition and his or her body weight, and is decided by a medical practitioner in many cases, or written on the container of drugs bought over the counter. Pharmacists will always respond to requests for clarification. Too low a dose of prescribed drugs can be as dangerous as too high a dose.

Drugs can be given

- by inhalation
- by injection
- by rubbing into the skin

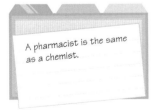

A pharmacist is the same as a chemist.

- by enema or suppository (inserted into the back passage)
- orally (which means by mouth).

Drugs should never be shared, and unused medication should be returned to the pharmacist.

Misuse of drugs intended as medical treatment

Some people become dependent on drugs originally prescribed for a limited length of time. Examples include sedatives prescribed to help people to sleep, tranquillisers to reduce anxiety, and stimulants to promote alertness.

Use of drugs with no accepted use in medical treatment

Drugs such as cannabis, heroin, cocaine, and ecstasy are not considered acceptable in western society. Their prolonged use is considered to be a danger to health and creates a dependency which is destructive to the abuser.

Misuse of solvents

Solvents are designed to strip paints, light cigarettes, fuel cars, and glue things together, not to be inhaled into people's lungs. Nevertheless, some people have a dependency on sniffing such substances, which causes confusion, loss of control, depression, and ultimately death of brain cells.

Misuse of drugs and solvents is always damaging, and can be fatal.

Good practice in maintaining hygiene

The two important aspects of hygiene to consider are **personal** and **public**.

Personal hygiene

Keeping clean requires some motivation and effort. People with low esteem, or a mental illness such as depression, find it hard to raise the energy to wash, bathe, and clean their clothes. Those who feel constantly tired or ill may give their personal hygiene a low priority. Often it is the most humble carer who looks after the cleanliness of clients. This is a very privileged position, as during baths, hair washing, or other intimate tasks a client will often talk freely and share their deepest thoughts, especially if the carer is scrupulous about attention to the client's privacy, dignity, and self-respect.

The aim of hygiene routines is to encourage people to be as clean as is needed for good health and to be as able as possible to maintain this level of cleanliness for themselves. The see-saw diagram on the following page looks at the objectives of personal hygiene and the potential barriers to achieving these.

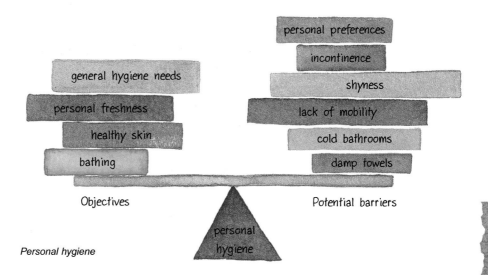

Objectives   Potential barriers

Personal hygiene

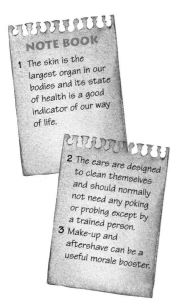

NOTE BOOK

1 The skin is the largest organ in our bodies and its state of health is a good indicator of our way of life.

2 The ears are designed to clean themselves and should normally not need any poking or probing except by a trained person.

3 Make-up and aftershave can be a useful morale booster.

People who are confused or psychologically damaged may cling to old routines. Older people may prefer the warm cosiness of a bath to the colder but quicker option of a shower. The use of deodorants may not be understood. Toenails may have become out of reach due to an expanding waistline or increasing joint stiffness. Moving about may be painful. If so, washing and dressing could be put off until after breakfast when the morning pain-killer may have been given and the body has had the chance to loosen up.

It is rare for clients not to be able to wash the intimate parts of their body themselves. If you do need to do this for them, be business-like and gentle, always paying attention to personal modesty – your own and the client's – and dignity. If you are performing a bed bath with a colleague, **never** make remarks or gestures that could be misinterpreted, even if your patient is unconscious. You can never tell what is being understood even when a person appears not to be aware – the sense of hearing is the last to leave a person's conscious mind.

All-over washing keeps the skin healthy and can be achieved by
- bathing
- showering
- strip washing (washing all over at a hand basin)
- bed bathing (washing all over while in bed)

Look for signs of dryness, rashes, and other skin abnormalities while you help people to wash.

Care of the hair means
- attention from a hairdresser
- washing
- trimming
- shaving
- removing unwanted hair
- dealing with head lice.

Care of the mouth means
- dental inspection
- a healthy diet
- brushing the teeth
- denture care
- keeping the mouth of an ill person fresh and clean.

Hygiene in public areas

Food hygiene

The **Food and Drugs Act 1955** and the **Food Hygiene (General) Regulations 1970** apply in all residential and nursing homes, and the manager is responsible for seeing that they are implemented. The basic rules will be displayed in the kitchen and should be followed by all staff.

Kitchen hygiene

The kitchen, both at home and at work, should be kept clean with hot soapy water, and tidied to reduce the risk of accidents. The table below gives a check list.

- Keep perishable food in a refrigerator.
- Clean the refrigerator regularly.
- Protect food from flies.
- Dispose of food scraps quickly.
- Use bins with lids and empty them frequently.
- Rinse out dishcloths and mops after use and leave to dry.

- Wash dishes in hot soapy water, rinse in hot water, and leave to drain. Then put them away in a cupboard or on a shelf.
- Wash up straight away or put dirty articles in the dishwasher rather than allow dirty dishes to pile up.

Eating areas

Dining areas, or personal trays, should be clean and attractive. Tray and table cloths will need washing often, as will table napkins if fabric ones are used. Cutlery should be shiny and crockery unchipped.

The floor will need sweeping or hoovering after each meal. Keep an eye open for tablets as these are often given out at mealtimes and may be unintentionally or intentionally dropped on to the floor.

Medical treatment areas

Medical treatment areas should be kept scrupulously clean. **Asepsis** means the absence of germs which can cause infection. It is impossible to achieve under normal conditions and therefore sterile

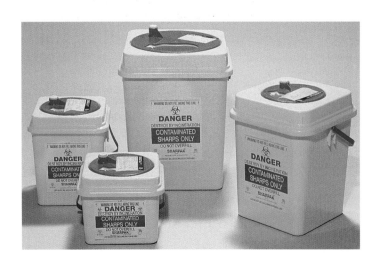

disposable dressings are used to cover wounds whenever aseptic conditions are required. In addition to a clean environment:

- all surfaces should be clean and dry and all staff should wash and dry their hands thoroughly, both before and after treatment

- after use, all disposable equipment should be wrapped up, put into a bag, and burnt

- sharp equipment should be put into a special yellow box labelled **'sharps'** and disposed of separately.

Safe practices in the workplace

The table below outlines factors to consider when ensuring that an environment is safe for individuals in different age groups. One particular environment that needs to be kept free of hazards is the workplace. Think about this in Activity D, question 6 (page 104).

Things to remember in looking after the safety of different groups of people

Crawlers and toddlers
- Never leave them alone where they could get into a dangerous situation.
- Remember that they can often move faster than you think.
- There is always the first time they begin to climb stairs.
- Look around to make sure everything hazardous is out of reach.
- They will listen to you because they trust you, but they are not able to understand rules.
- Their curiosity gets them into trouble.
- Keep a close eye on them in the garden.
- Teach them safe habits.

Children over 5 years old
- You will not always be with them – they need to develop independence.
- Talk to them often about the dangers they may meet. At this age they should have some understanding of accidents and danger.
- Set them a good example – they will imitate you more readily than they listen to you.
- Let them cook under supervision so they will learn safe habits.
- Encourage them to be tidy.
- Never let them swim alone.
- They are not safe alone on the road. Teach them the Green Cross Code.
- Make sure they learn how to behave safely when travelling in a car – seat belts fastened, not distracting the driver.

Older children
- By the time they are old enough to be independent, children need to have learnt safe habits of behaviour.
- Teach them to be in control of their own safety.
- Discuss with them what to do in an emergency.
- Make sure they have proper instruction if they want to take part in dangerous activities.
- Only allow them on the road alone after they are 10 years old, or older, depending on their personality and abilities.
- Give them road safety training.
- Make sure they wear cycling helmets.
- Encourage them to learn how to maintain cycles in a good, safe condition.
- They must be visible on the road, during the day and after dark.

Adults
- Young adults are more likely to take **calculated risks**. They understand the risks, but expect to 'get away' with dangerous behaviour, such as running across roads, cycling in a risky way, driving a little too fast.
- Older adults tend to be wiser, as their own and their friends' experience may have taught them that dangers and accidents are very real.

Elderly people
- may not recognise their increasing frailty and loss of co-ordination.
- may not see and hear as well as they used to.
- may have thrifty habits which restrict their use of lighting and heating.
- may have homes which need repair and maintenance which have been overlooked.
- have bones which break more easily.
- may fall because of increasing infirmity or illness.

unit two

ACTIVITY D

1 Examine the table on page 103.

2 List the main hazards to which adults are exposed.

3 Identify the hazards that each of the age groups may be exposed to during different recreational activities.

4 Describe how each of the hazards might affect their health.

5 Describe how the hazards might be reduced. **C2.3**

6 Repeat steps 3 to 5, this time looking at client risk in work settings. You could use the four described in the case studies.

7 Make a floor plan of your work room at school or college, marking on it where there are potential safety hazards.

◆▶ **Extension opportunity**

Find some statistics for accidents in the age groups concerned. Present them in a suitable format. Explain how you checked the validity of the data.

How stress affects health and well-being

The table below outlines the possible effects of stress. Responses to stress vary in strength and duration depending on the individuals concerned and their stages of development, and on the significance to them of the causes of the stress.

Small children and people who cannot express themselves are especially likely to show their responses through their behaviour. It is important for carers to understand this, as changed habits may be explained by some underlying stress in the individual's personal life.

The four lists in the table suggest that the effects of stress are always bad. However, stress can act as a positive stimulus which will then affect individuals in a helpful way.

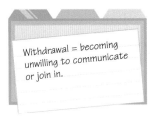

Withdrawal = becoming unwilling to communicate or join in.

Possible effects of stress

1. Effects on emotional life	2. Effects on social life
Withdrawal	Not getting out of bed
Outburst of temper	Staying at home, away from work or school
Unable to relate to people	Not coming home at night
Loss of trust	Not wanting to go out
Low self-esteem	Change of habits
	Change in language and speech

3. Effects on intellectual activity	4. Effects on physical habits
Loss of motivation	Change in eating habits
Becoming workaholic (working too hard)	Altered sleep patterns
Regression (children going back a stage)	Hyperactivity
Low attention span (cannot concentrate for long)	Weight loss or gain
Mental illness	Eating disorders (anorexia, bulimia)
Depression	Regression (thumb sucking, bed-wetting)
	Rocking or head banging
	Violence
	Drug or alcohol abuse

ACTIVITY E

1 Think about two stressful situations you have experienced, one which you felt bad about, one which you felt good about.

2 Make a list of the effects each of them had on you.

3 Sort these effects into four categories – emotional, social, intellectual, and physical. You will find that the effects overlap and relate to one another in complex ways.

Social class

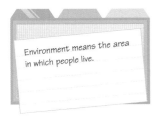

Environment means the area in which people live.

Traditionally, the main access to opportunities is through occupation, and this has become the principal way of dividing people into social classes, although class divisions are really far more complex than this. Social class determines social factors like environment, employment, housing, income, and education, each of which has an influence on people's health and well-being, as shown in the following tables.

Aspects of the five social factors

unit two

1 Environment

Aspects to consider:

a suburban means on the outskirts of the town

b rural means in the countryside
  • high travel costs to work
  • homes may be rented or owner-occupied.
  • access to shops, community, friends, and family

c urban means in towns
  • ability to buy own house
  • restricted amount of available rented accommodation
  • low travel costs to work.
  • restriction by local authority residence requirements

d inner cities mainly concern Birmingham, Liverpool, Manchester, Newcastle, and areas of London
  • created by massive population increase in the nineteenth century
  • density of population remains, properties are old and need renovating
  • absentee landlords may not want to spend money on improvements
  • shared accommodation in different storeys
  • elderly people not wishing to renovate
  • access, congestion, and crime may discourage the creation of new job opportunities.
  • many demands on social and health services

Some inner-city areas develop a village-like culture which makes life for its residents more community-oriented and settled.

2 Employment

Aspects to consider:
  • inner-city addresses can influence job selection
  • distance and cost of transport to work each day
  • language
  • culture
  • ambition
  • education
  • qualifications
  • motivation
  • family responsibilities
  • other demands on energy, emotions, finances

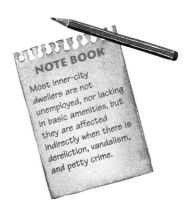

NOTE BOOK

Most inner-city dwellers are not unemployed, nor lacking in basic amenities, but they are affected indirectly when there is dereliction, vandalism, and petty crime.

3 Housing

Aspects to consider:

- owner-occupied (lived in by the owner who has bought outright or can pay a mortgage)
- rented (from someone on the premises or living away – 'absentee landlord')
- detached
- semi-detached
- terraced
- a house
- a bungalow
- a flat
- a maisonette
- have a garden
- do not have a garden
- travelling people moving from place to place
- no settled address

4 Income

Aspects to consider:

- low-income elderly
- low-income families
- lowest skilled/least well paid
- low-income groups are most prone to ill health
- immigrants may not understand how to gain access to benefits or apply for work
- people earning more money than they need for day-to-day living have disposable income, which means that they have spare money they can spend on holidays, treats, house improvements, and investment.
- the opposite is true of low-income families

This can lead to

- an upward spiral of increased success for those with a reasonable income and access to opportunity.
- a downward spiral of poverty for those with a low income and few opportunities.

5 Education

Aspects to consider:

- encourages the learning of basic skills of reading and numeracy
- passes on social patterns of behaviour from one generation to the next
- prepares people for work
- ethnic groups – language difficulties affect education of children/communication with parents
- situation of schools
- type of school
  public
  private
  state
  boarding or day
  single sex or co-educational
  selective (i.e. grammar) or comprehensive
  age based   – nursery up to the age of 5
          – primary 5–11
          – secondary 11–16 or 18
          – further education (FE) 16–18
          – higher education (HE) 18 up
          – adult education
- qualifications currently available
  Post-16 = GCSE, GNVQ, A level and equivalent, graduate
  Higher education = degree or equivalent, or non-graduate qualifications gained at HE institutions.
  Boundaries are blurred as establishments franchise and widen the selection of courses they offer.

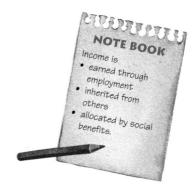

NOTE BOOK

Income is
- earned through employment
- inherited from others
- allocated by social benefits.

The possible impact of social factors on individual choices which affect health and well-being

Social factors have an enormous impact on people's lives, yet are often outside their control. People's way of life is affected by where they live, how much money they have, whether they have a job or not, and their qualifications. These factors decide how much **choice** there is about lifestyle, health, and well-being.

Individual choices

Most people have some degree of choice in the following areas of their lives:

- using health and care services
- nutrition
- alcohol consumption
- smoking habits
- personal hygiene
- exercise
- attitude to education
- maintenance of housing/accommodation
- use of available income – that is, how spending is planned.

ACTIVITY F

1 Make a chart showing the relationship between the five *factors* (environment, employment, housing, income, and education) and the four *choices* (health, attitude to education, maintenance of housing, and use of available income).

2 Use the following scale to indicate the effect of the factors on the choices: 1 = low impact, 2 = medium impact, 3 = high impact.

3 Discuss with your colleagues how these choices could affect or have an impact on individuals' health and well-being.

unit two

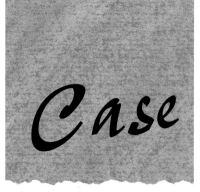

Case Studies

Case study 2.1　The Thatched Cottage

Eileen is a recent arrival. Before admission, she lived alone in a cold flat, not eating properly, and having no inclination to wash or change her clothes. She enjoys it in The Thatched Cottage, being warm and having her food prepared for her. She snoozes comfortably in an armchair most of the day.

She is now finding it difficult to sleep through the night and is beginning to put on weight. She admits she is becoming lazy about hygiene, but 'can't see the point' now that she is no longer responsible for her own washing and cleaning. She has agreed to help Mark with his college coursework.

Before you start, make a reference list of

a the most important reasons for following a balanced way of life

b methods of reducing health risks

c the effects of substance and drug abuse on health and well-being (from Activity C, page 99).

Then, using the information you have gathered together, respond to the case studies presented here.

Task 1

1　How could Mark work out what might have happened to the balance of Eileen's lifestyle which would cause these changes?

2　How might he demonstrate this with a before and after see-saw?

3　How could he explain to Eileen why a balanced lifestyle is important?

Task 1

4　What are the most important aspects of good practice in personal hygiene which might help to motivate Eileen?

5　Using images – drawn either by hand or using a computer – explain the importance of hygienic practices in one of the public areas of The Thatched Cottage.

IT2.1, 2.2, 2.3

Case study 2.2　Down Way School

Kevin is five, and has asthma. An inhaler is kept in the staff room for him to use before he plays football, which he loves and plays very well. When Jalwinder hangs up his coat one day it smells strongly of stale cigarette smoke. Three empty crisp packets fall out of the pockets, which could explain why Kevin eats so little at lunch time.

Task 2

Write a report in which you consider the following issues:

1　If she had to discuss his health with his parents, how would Jalwinder explain the following

C2.3

Task 2

a　why the school thinks it is important for him to continue to play football

b　the effect of cigarette smoke on his state of health

c　other ways of reducing health risks in general.

Case study 2.3   Netherfield Community Care

Debbie's aunt, who works in the local doctor's surgery, knows that Debbie is following a course in Health and Social Care. She becomes friendly with Jane, a patient who has ME (Myalgic encephalomyelitis, which causes severe fatigue over a long period of time), and is pregnant. She wants to help Jane to eat well during her pregnancy, and is also concerned that James, Jane's young son, should eat sensibly. Jane's grandmother lives next door, and often gives James sweets and chocolates.

Debbie's aunt suggests that Debbie should make out a list for Jane of the foods which would be of benefit to her, James, and her grandmother. The list is to help with the shopping, and also with a typical day's menu for all three individuals. Jane is interested to know why each of the foods recommended is good for their health, and how much of it they should eat.

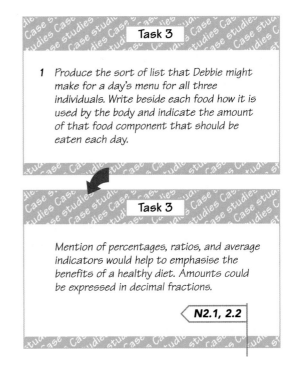

Task 3

1   Produce the sort of list that Debbie might make for a day's menu for all three individuals. Write beside each food how it is used by the body and indicate the amount of that food component that should be eaten each day.

Task 3

Mention of percentages, ratios, and average indicators would help to emphasise the benefits of a healthy diet. Amounts could be expressed in decimal fractions.

N2.1, 2.2

Case study 2.4   Hill Hall

Many of the children are dependent on medication to make their lives tolerable. Danny is a new boy. His mother has become interested in herbal remedies and wants to discuss discontinuing his prescribed drugs and substituting others which her daughter finds helpful. The staff are talking about this over coffee. Some sympathise with the mother's view, others disagree with her.

Task 4

Discuss in a group

a   how prescribed drugs might be helping Danny

b   possible results of discontinuing them

c   with whom it would be appropriate for Danny's mother to discuss the changes she desires

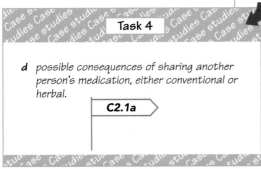

Task 4

d   possible consequences of sharing another person's medication, either conventional or herbal.

C2.1a

unit two **case studies**

Multiple Choice Questions

2.1 Which person has the greatest need of protein in the diet?

   a   *an eight-year-old child*

   b   *a middle-aged man*

   c   *an elderly woman*

   d   *a thirty-year-old woman*

2.2 Which of the following is *most* likely to be affected by inadequate body hygiene?

   a   *dietary intake*

   b   *intellectual development*

   c   *personal activities*

   d   *physical health*

2.3 When a person spends a long time sitting down, his or her lifestyle is described as being

   a   *passive*

   b   *mobile*

   c   *sedentary*

   d   *active*

2.4 Decide which of these statements about food is true (T) and which is false (F).

   a   *plenty of salt is good for you*

   b   *fibre makes you fat*

   c   *food can be a substitute for love*

   d   *you feel less hungry for longer after eating potatoes than after eating sweets*

   e   *people should drink less as they grow older*

2.5 Drug abuse means that

   a   *vitamin supplements are taken unnecessarily*

   b   *tranquillisers are taken regularly*

   c   *prescribed drugs are taken in recommended doses*

   d   *drugs are taken which have no accepted use in medical treatment*

2.6 Which of the following is a health risk?

   a   *a vegetarian eating beans instead of meat*

   b   *a housewife drinking a glass of red wine each evening*

   c   *a person with diabetes taking less insulin than the prescribed dose*

   d   *a child climbing a tree*

2.7 Fats in the diet are used by the body to

   a   *repair tissues*

   b   *provide energy*

   c   *convert glucose*

   d   *prevent constipation*

2.8 Which *one* of the following phrases *best* describes a balanced diet?

   a   *food is eaten only when a person is hungry*

   b   *adequate protein is taken to repair damaged cells*

   c   *all food components are taken in adequate quantities*

   d   *food intake is sufficient to maintain body weight*

CROSSWORD 'Food for thought'

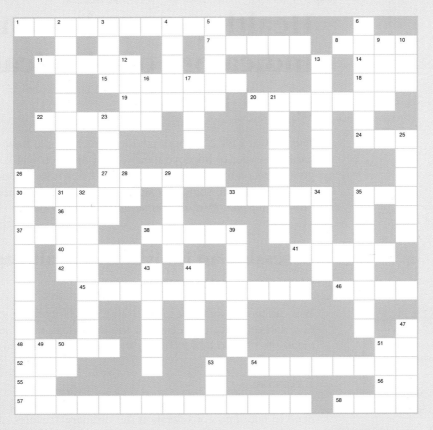

Across

1 Naughty but nice   5, 5
7 What you pay for food   5
8 Not recommended in excess   4
11 Sooner or later it may settle on the bottom!   5
14 A star sign   3
15 Contains nicotine   7
18 It contains preserved food   3
19 Families eat their meals from it   5
20 The body builder   7
22 Description of someone whose religion prohibits the eating of pork   6
24 Does it gather germs in the sink?   3
27 We shouldn't do this between meals   6
30 Do they keep the doctor away?   6
33 A mother does this when she gets her baby used to solid food   5
35 None on food   3
36 Meat less good for you than white   3
37 Comes from cows   4
38 Angry action for teeth?   5
40 A way to fry   4
41 Someone who eats no animal products   5
42 Thus   2

45 People who eat no meat   11
46 Can be made from sunflowers, nuts and olives   4
48 Not quite right   5
51 Fourth note of scale   2
52 Green bottles?   3
54 6 down is one of the essential ones   8
55 A prefix   2
56 Describes position   2
57 Types of 26 down   5, 3, 6
58 We cook in them   4

Down

2 Code letters for additives   1, 7
3 Source of animal protein   4
4 Turkish way of serving food   5
5 Variety is the – – – – – of life   5
6 Essential for strong teeth and bones   7
9 Contains little fat   4
10 A measure of weight seldom used in cooking!   3
12 Food does this if not kept cool in hot weather   4
13 Lancashire stew   6
16 Expression of disgust   3

17 Can result from hardening of the arteries   4
21 Is now known as fibre   8
23 Pressed   6
25 Causes jam to set   6
26 Give us energy   13
28 State of being   2
29 Runners, jumping or black eyed!   5
31 Squeeze   5
32 Eating too many puts on weight   4-5
34 Does the thought of mint sauce frighten them?   5
35 Supplements not always necessary   8
39 State of cleanliness desirable in the kitchen   7
43 Source of vegetable protein   6
44 Food provided   4
47 Doesn't eat   5
49 Bill of fare   4
50 Contained   2
51 An open tart   4
53 Essential for health – but don't eat too much   3

Unit 2.3
Health promotion and indicators of physical good health

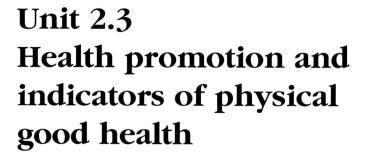

This part of Unit 2 is about advising other people how to adapt their habits in order to improve their way of life. You will learn about the general recommendations currently laid down for good health, so that you have definite standards against which you can measure someone's present lifestyle. This, of course, includes your own.

Assessing an individual's health against standard measures

You can assess someone's health in terms of exercise, diet, sleep and rest, and other factors related to the individual, using standard measures of food tables, fitness measures, and physical measures.

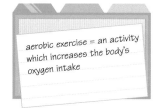

aerobic exercise = an activity which increases the body's oxygen intake

Exercise

When working out how much exercise a person takes each day, we need to take into consideration the ordinary activities of his or her daily life: for instance, walking upstairs, walking to the shops or work, cycling, housework, looking after a toddler, gardening, or operating a wheelchair or frame. All of these help to keep the heart and lungs healthy, which is called **cardiovascular fitness**. An increase in everyday activities is to be encouraged before someone is recommended to take up a sport. It can be harmful for an unfit person to undertake sudden strenuous activity.

The benefits of being fit are felt after any increase in exercise, such as walking, cycling, jogging, dancing, swimming, badminton, or football. All of these are examples of **aerobic exercise**, which is the most beneficial for cardiovascular fitness.

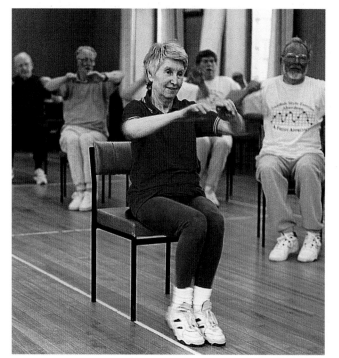

People who have recovered from a heart attack attend an exercise class at the hospital, to help build up their fitness.

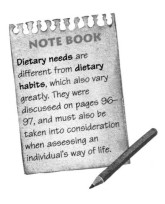

Diet

People's dietary needs vary greatly according to

- age – young children need more protein than adults
- mode of life – active or sedentary
- state of health
- personal metabolism – the rate at which energy is burned up
- personal dietary needs – people may need a special diet to keep them in good health, for example, those with diabetes.

Sleep and rest, and relaxation

Individual needs for sleep vary; babies sleep a great deal, gradually requiring less sleep as they grow older. Older people generally sleep less than young adults. The table below shows the average number of hours of sleep needed by different age groups.

Average hours of sleep needed

New born baby	20 hours	Adult	8 hours
Infant	12 hours	Older person	7 hours
Child	10 hours		

At all ages individual needs vary according to temperament and level of physical activity.

As we grow older we tend to sleep less, but our need for relaxation and rest increases. Young children need opportunities to recover from running about and other physical activities necessary to the healthy development of their bodies. Everybody needs relaxation for the mind and brain to recover from mental and emotional activities.

Factors related to the individual

All the following will affect people's inclination or ability to act on advice about their general level of health:

- general health and level of fitness
- presence of illness
  - short-term (e.g. measles)
  - long-term (e.g. asthma)
- mental health (for example, the client may be schizophrenic)
- level of understanding (for example, the client may be autistic)
- gender and age – women tend to respond to health advice more readily than men. Younger men tend to respond to health advice more readily than older men.

unit two

Standard measures of health

People's health can be assessed by comparing their diet, fitness levels, and weight with various standard measures. For example, an individual's diet can be compared with the diet recommended by the Department of Health shown below.

Food tables

Food tables like this are one example of a standard measure of health.

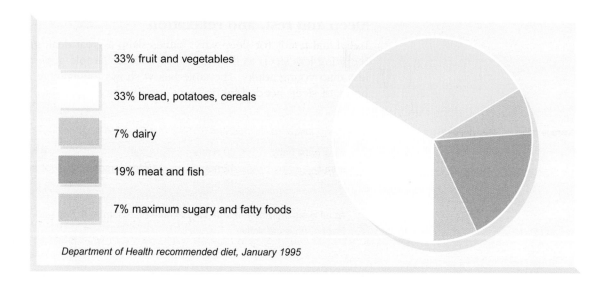

33% fruit and vegetables

33% bread, potatoes, cereals

7% dairy

19% meat and fish

7% maximum sugary and fatty foods

Department of Health recommended diet, January 1995

ACTIVITY A

1 Take your own pulse (at the wrist or the neck) when you have not been active for some time. Also take the pulse of a friend.

2 Take your pulses again, after you have both done some exercise (e.g. running on the spot for one minute; climbing stairs)

3 Show the information in a table. Then present it in a graph.

> *N2.1, 2.3*

Fitness measures

A person's pulse rate is a good indicator of their heart and circulation fitness. Checking a person's pulse against a chart like the one on the next page gives you an indication of their fitness level.

Taking the pulse at the wrist

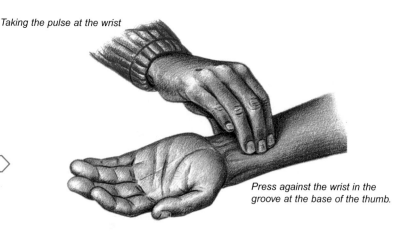

Press against the wrist in the groove at the base of the thumb.

Analysis of average pulse rates

	Resting			After activity *		
Age group	*Young*	*Middle*	*Elderly*	*Young*	*Middle*	*Elderly*
Men						
Good	60 – 70	65 – 72	68 – 75	76 – 84	80 – 88	84 – 90
Average	71 – 85	73 – 87	76 – 90	85 – 100	89 – 104	91 – 104
Poor	86+	88+	91+	101+	105+	105+
Women						
Good	72 – 77	72 – 79	77 – 83	88 – 92	88 – 94	92 – 98
Average	78 – 95	80 – 98	84 – 102	93 – 110	95 – 114	99 – 116
Poor	96+	99+	103+	111+	115+	117+

* For example, running on the spot for 1 minute.

Safe maximum pulse rate		
Age group	*Young*	*Middle*	*Elderly*
	170	155	140

The pulse should not exceed these rates during exercise.

unit two

Another measure of a person's fitness is their **lung efficiency**. Activity B looks at measuring lung efficiency without the need for a peak flow meter.

Measuring 'peak flow' means measuring the maximum volume of air that can be exhaled or inhaled in one minute. This is usually expressed as **Peak Expiratory Flow**, or PEF, and it is an indicator of how well the breathing muscles and the respiratory tract are working. A special piece of equipment, called a peak flow meter, with a disposable mouthpiece, is used, and the best of three measures is taken as the client's record. Normal peak flow varies according to the gender and height of the person involved. Tall men have greater lung capacity than short women.

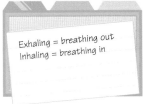

Exhaling = breathing out
Inhaling = breathing in

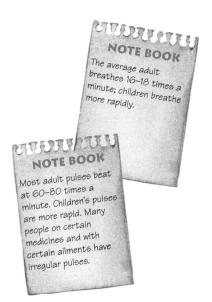

NOTE BOOK
The average adult breathes 16–18 times a minute; children breathe more rapidly.

NOTE BOOK
Most adult pulses beat at 60–80 times a minute. Children's pulses are more rapid. Many people on certain medicines and with certain ailments have irregular pulses.

ACTIVITY B

How efficient are your lungs?

1 Time how long you can hold your breath – it should be 45 seconds or more.

2 Measure your chest when you have breathed in and again after breathing out. The difference should be 5–7 cms.

These measures can be used with clients to see if breathing exercises would improve their lung capacity.

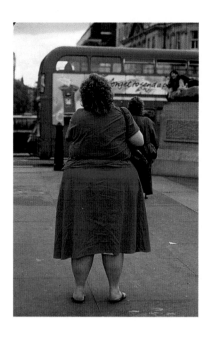

Physical measures

Weight and **body fat** are useful physical measures. In 1999 it was estimated that 30–35% of the UK population carried too much weight and that about 5% were obese.

The standard measure of weight is the **body mass index**, or BMI. To work out your body mass index, you take your weight in kilograms and divide it by the square of your height in metres.

$$BMI = \frac{weight\ (kg)}{height\ (m) \times height\ (m)}$$

A BMI of 30 or more means you are dangerously overweight, or **obese**.

A BMI of 25–30 means you are overweight.

The table below shows recommended height/weight ratios as advised by the Health Education Authority.

Recommended height/weight ratios (Health Education Authority)

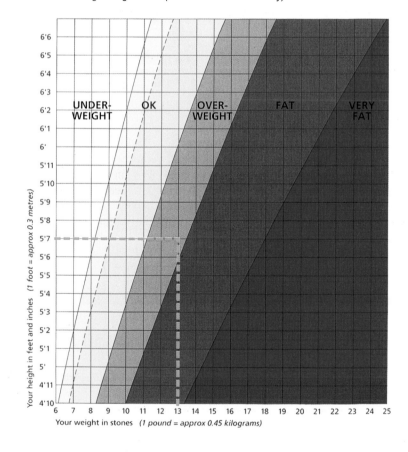

ACTIVITY C

1 Measure the height and weight of a range of people.

2 Present the information using a variety of graphical methods.

3 Summarise the information displayed by using appropriate representative values – e.g. median.

4 Measure the BMI **N2.1, 2.2, 2.3** of each individual, showing your calculations.

5 Enter this information into a spreadsheet and select an appropriate graphing method to display it – e.g. pie chart, bar chart.

IT2.1, 2.2, 2.3

ACTIVITY D

Working in pairs:

1 Breathe out and relax.

2 Measure waist.

3 Breathe in.

4 Measure chest when lungs are full.

5 Work out the difference between the two
measurements, displaying
all numerical calculations **N2.1, 2.2, 2.3**
when reaching conclusions
drawn from results.

If the waist measurement is greater than the chest
measurement, there is a need to lose weight.

◀▶ Extension opportunity

1 Think about a person you know well, who feels
that their personal health or well-being would
benefit from attention.

2 Find some standard measure(s) of health and well-
being other than those explained above, which
would be relevant to this person.

3 Assess the individual's health against the
measure(s).

4 Make a record of the procedure you have
undertaken. Remember the confidentiality issues.

If you are able to gain the person's consent and
approval, you could make this a real exercise.

unit two

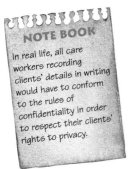

NOTE BOOK

In real life, all care workers recording clients' details in writing would have to conform to the rules of confidentiality in order to respect their clients' rights to privacy.

Producing a plan to improve an individual's health

Now that you have learnt some of the ways of measuring an
individual's state of health, you will learn how to draw up a plan to
help someone to lead a more healthy life. The starting-point must be
an assessment of the person's present state of health, from which you
devise an action plan.

The action plan

An action plan needs to consider the priorities for action – that is, the
order of importance of the different things that need improving. The
personal targets that the client hopes to achieve in the short and long
term need to be thought through. Later, at the appraisal stage, these
targets need to be reassessed. Do they need to be changed?

ACTIVITY E

Continue with case study 2.2, about Kevin at
Down Way School (page 108).

1 Using the table on pages 118-119 as a model,
but adapting it where you feel necessary,
draw up an assessment for Kevin.

2 Devise an action plan from your findings.

ACTIVITY F

1 Working in pairs, draw up an action plan for
each of you, showing your estimate of where
you need to improve your personal health.

2 Decide when your targets should be
reviewed. Don't attempt too many changes.
Your plan needs to be realistic.

Plan for living

1 Assessment

Name ....   Date ....

a Present state of health   *Good*   *Acceptable*   *Poor*   *Good*   *Acceptable*   *Poor*

	Good	Acceptable	Poor		Good	Acceptable	Poor
Physical fitness				*Taking of prescribed*			
Diet				*medication (if applicable)*			
Hygiene				*Rest/relaxation*			
Smoking				*Substance abuse*			
Alcohol consumption				*Drug dependency*			

Anything appearing in the *'poor'* column needs carrying on to chart b.
You will guess that some of the topics will need tactful discussion.

b Risks to health

Level of risk	No risk	Low - not dangerous			High - dangerous	
	0	1	2	3	4	5
Level of physical exercise						
Diet						
Hygiene						
Smoking						
Alcohol consumption						
Taking of prescribed medication (if applicable)						
Rest/relaxation						
Substance abuse						
Drug dependency						

c Factors to be considered (circle as applicable)

General health	*Good*	*Average*	*Poor*	*if poor, explain*

Presence of illness   short-term   state cause ....

                              long-term   state cause ....

Mental health   *Good*   *Average*   *Poor*   *if poor, explain*

Level of understanding *explain*

2 Action plan

Things which need to be improved	Ways of improving them	Order of importance

Targets   What the client hopes to achieve: What the benefits will be:

a short-term

b long-term

Appraisal
Have the things in the first list improved?
Do the targets need to be changed?
If so, in what way?

Date

Producing and presenting advice on maintaining health and well-being related to the needs of a target group

Carers often have to give health advice to groups of those they look after. These are called **target groups** and could be any of the following:

- children
- pregnant women
- elderly people
- those who are physically active
- those who are sedentary
- people with physical disabilities.

Sometimes individuals fit into more than one group.

We need to know which target group individuals fit into so that any health advice given can be set out in a way which is suitable for them. Otherwise it will not be understood or acted upon. The way advice is presented is called its **presentation format**.

ACTIVITY G

1 Into which target groups would the clients in case studies 2.1-2.4 fit? (See pages 108-109.)

2 Record your findings.

*Choose an appropriate method:
Written – booklet or leaflet?
Pictorial – poster, photo, cartoon,
computer graphic?
Diagrammatic – bar chart, pie
chart, graph?
Tape recorder?
Video?*

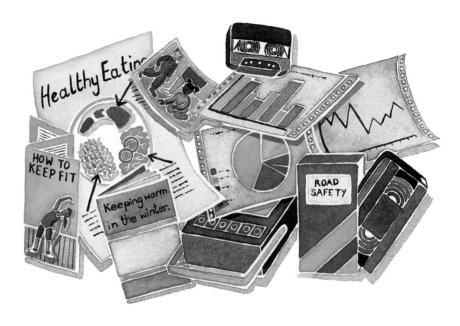

*Choose a sensible system:
right language, right order, right
contents, right colour and style.*

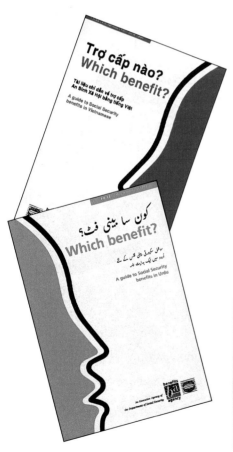

Choices of presentation format

1 **Written** – will only work when the clients can read and understand the writing.

2 **Diagrammatic** – sometimes conveys the meaning more clearly than words.

3 **Pictorial** – it has been said that a picture saves a thousand words: sometimes a picture is more attractive than writing, and often it is easier to understand.

4 **Audio-visual** – a good way to transmit complicated information and often suitable for groups.

The tables below show some of the design choices that need to be made, and some practical points that will affect the choices you make.

DESIGN CHOICES	PRACTICAL POINTS
• size and type of paper • use of colour • medium – paint, crayon, felt pen, etc. • amount of space on the page • colour of background • best layout – poster, booklet, leaflet, etc.	• cost • availability of material • skills of team (if applicable) • own abilities • distribution of finished presentation • time constraints

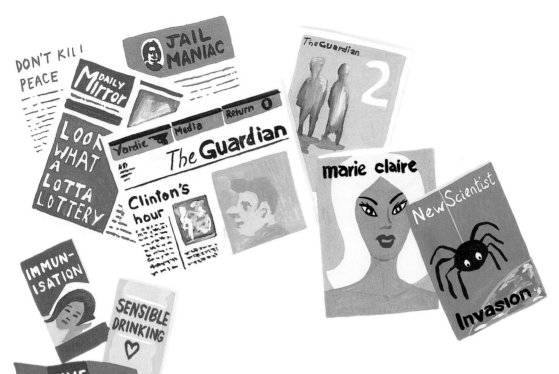

Make sure of your information
Is it up-to-date? reliable? accurate?
Did I get it from a source I can trust?
Do I need to check it?

Assessing the impact of the advice on the target group

After any work with clients, it is wise to spend time looking back to see how useful the activity has been. This is called **evaluation**. In this case you want to discover how effective your presentation has been, and whether or not your clients have acted on the advice you gave. Sometimes the effort seems to have no effect, and often the effect is difficult to measure, especially if the target group finds it hard to put thoughts into words because they are too young, too old, or too disabled to describe things using words.

Evaluation is carried out by getting **feedback** from the clients. You need to find out if the presentation format was appropriate, and if they intend to take notice of the information it contained.

This can be done by formal or informal methods.

Formal methods

Formal methods can take the form of a series of questions with responses. The responses could be

- **verbal** – for example, a group discussion for formal review
- **written** – for example, a simple tick or cross, 'smiley' faces showing degrees of pleasure and displeasure, or graded numbers.

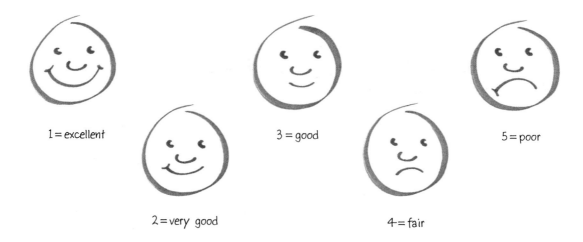

Informal methods

More informal methods of evaluation include

- watching behaviour
- asking questions
- seeing if habits change
- listening for comments
- informal discussion.

The skill lies in selecting a method which can be easily used and understood by the client group involved. You will also have to decide whether your findings need to be recorded and/or reported to others.

Case Studies

Case study 3.1   Hill Hall

There are four people with moderate learning difficulties living semi-independently in an annexe to Hill Hall school. It is suspected that someone has been climbing in over the wall and inhaling solvents in the back garden during the night. The residents are impressionable, so there is a danger that they could find and experiment with the debris that is left, or try to copy the habit. Molly discovers that Ann enjoys planning projects, and realises that this is an opportunity to help her to communicate with the clients in a very useful way.

Task 1

1   Molly asks Ann to design a health promotion package explaining to the residents of the hostel the dangers of substance abuse. Use the information in the text to help you decide on an appropriate presentation format.

Task 1

Then design the package that Ann might produce. The format should NOT be a poster – you will be using this in Case study 3.3. You may decide to use a computer for this activity.

IT2.1, 2.2, 2.3 ⟩

Task 1

2   How might Ann devise an appropriate method of evaluating the effectiveness of her advice?

Case study 3.2   The Thatched Cottage

Dora is going to aerobics classes and is feeling very fit and well. She wants to share her enthusiasm with the residents by encouraging them to take more exercise within their capabilities. She enlists Mark's help with some suitable music on his tape recorder, and the residents begin gentle exercises in their chairs.

Task 2

1   How could Dora and Mark work out the effectiveness of their scheme?

2   How long should they wait before assessing its value, and why?

123

Case study 3.3 Netherfield Community Care

Several young men live together in a hostel for people with physical disabilities. Different aids to mobility allow them to keep active, their kitchen is adapted for cooking, and they shop for one another in a nearby shopping precinct. They have asked Debbie and Mikhail to produce a poster to explain to them realistic ways of reducing health risks in their daily lives. They want it to look good as it is intended for their sitting room.

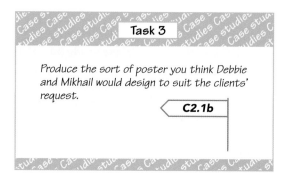

Task 3

Produce the sort of poster you think Debbie and Mikhail would design to suit the clients' request.

C2.1b

Case study 3.4 Down Way School

Some of the children have been eating reluctantly at lunchtime. It is found that they have seen a television programme about reducing diets, and they have decided to slim. Isabel and Jalwinder want to do some work with the children about healthy eating and appropriate height/weight ratios for their age. The aim is to strengthen the work the teaching staff are doing with the parents about the children's lunches.

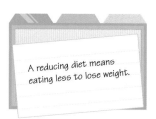

A reducing diet means eating less to lose weight.

Task 4

1 What standard measures of health might Isabel and Jalwinder use with the children?
2 How could they make this interesting for the children?

Task 4

3 In what way would the presentation be different from, and in what ways would it be similar to, presentations appropriate for the other three work placements?

Task 4

4 How could the findings be recorded?
5 How could Isabel and Jalwinder find out the children's immediate response to their advice?

Write up your opinions with examples.

Multiple Choice Questions

3.1 Working out the state of a person's health is called

   a *acceptability*

   b *accreditation*

   c *assessment*

   d *evaluation*

3.2 Which of the following is a standard measure of health?

   a *protein/carbohydrate ratio*

   b *height/weight ratio*

   c *health/fitness ratio*

   d *sleep/relaxation ratio*

3.3 After carrying out a health promotion exercise, which of the following would show that your advice had been ignored?

   a *the client's habits would remain unchanged*

   b *the client's health would improve*

   c *the carers would feel less stressed*

   d *the carers' relations with the client would improve*

3.4 When things are prioritised, they are

   a *left unfinished*

   b *put in alphabetical order*

   c *put in order of importance*

   d *done immediately*

3.5 Which would be the *most* suitable method of promoting care of the teeth to a class of five-year-old children?

   a *a typed page of information*

   b *a formal lecture*

   c *a written quiz*

   d *a cartoon poster*

3.6 When assessing an elderly man's lifestyle, it is discovered that he enjoys late-night television programmes. Which of the following effects would be considered a health risk?

   a *it causes him to go to bed late*

   b *it stops him from sleeping well*

   c *his wife disapproves*

   d *he seldom watches day-time television*

See also questions 3.7 and 3.8 on the next page.

Note: These questions are for you to test your knowledge. There is no formal multiple choice test in this GNVQ.

unit two

Multiple Choice Questions

3.7 Which of these pie charts illustrates best the recommended dietary components?

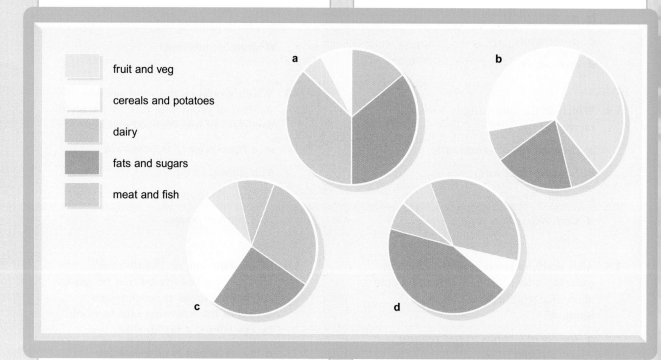

fruit and veg

cereals and potatoes

dairy

fats and sugars

meat and fish

a

b

c

d

◆ **Extension opportunity**
You could record and present the pie charts in approximate percentages, fractions, or decimal fractions.

3.8 Which *one* of the following could be described as a long-term personal target for inclusion in a health plan?

a *maintaining an exercise programme*

b *assessing the individual's lifestyle*

c *evaluating the effects of the plan*

d *identifying priorities for action*

Note: These questions are for you to test your knowledge. There is no formal multiple choice test in this GNVQ.

Compulsory Assessment Activity

Evidence for Unit Two

Here is an outline of the main evidence you are required to produce in order to be successful in Unit Two. The optional tasks and activities described throughout the unit chapter (pages 86-126) have been designed to make it easier for you to complete this final compulsory piece of work. Your teaching staff need to approve your chosen topic, so the following information intentionally gives only broad guidance.

You must produce a plan for promoting health and well-being for at least one person who is at risk. The plan must include

- information about the risks to health, identifying those over which the individual(s) may have control

- at least two measures of health

- timescales and targets for improvement

- supporting health promotion materials.

In order to achieve a pass, you must show that you can

- understand the factors that affect the health and well-being of your chosen person, by considering physical factors and at least one social and emotional factor (see page 93, *Factors affecting health and well-being*)

- explain clearly factors which cause potential risks to the health and well-being of your chosen person (see page 93, *Factors affecting health and well-being*)

- correctly use and interpret the measures you have chosen (see page 112, *Health promotion and indicators of physical good health*)

- communicate your plan in a form appropriate to your chosen person and explain clearly how the targets can be met (see page 112, *Health promotion and indicators of physical good health*)

- clearly explain why the health promotion materials were selected (see page 112, *Health promotion and indicators of physical good health*).

If you are keen to gain a merit or distinction, your work will need to be more complex. Your teacher or lecturer will tell you how to achieve these higher grades.

unit two

Summary of evidence opportunities

2.1 How to define health and well-being

Activity A (page 88)

Case studies 1.1, 1.2, 1.3 (pages 90-91)

2.2 Factors affecting health and well-being

Activities A (page 95), B (page 98), C (page 99), D (page 104)

Case studies 2.1, 2.2, 2.3, 2.4 (pages 108-109)

2.3 Health promotion and indicators of physical good health

Activities A (page 114), B (page 115), C (page 116), D (page 117), E (page 117), F (page 117), G (page 119)

Case studies 3.1, 3.2, 3.3, 3.4 (pages 123-124)

Personal evidence tracking record

Remember that you can use portfolio evidence more than once, to show understanding of other units.

2.1 How to define health and well-being	Description of evidence	Portfolio reference number
Physical aspects		
Social aspects		
Intellectual aspects		
Emotional aspects		
Health and well-being in:		
infants		
young children		
adolescents		
adults		
elderly people		

2.2 Factors affecting health and well-being		
Diet, exercise, and recreation		
Environment		
Social class		
Employment		
Housing		
Income		
Education		
Risk factors		
substance abuse		
diet		
stress		
poor personal hygiene		
lack of physical exercise		
unsafe sexual behaviour		
unsafe practices in the workplace		

unit two

2.3 Health promotion and indicators of physical good health	Description of evidence	Portfolio reference number
Producing health targets		
Using physical measures of health		
height and weight		
peak flow		
body mass index		
resting pulse and recovery after exercise		
Negotiating health improvement targets		

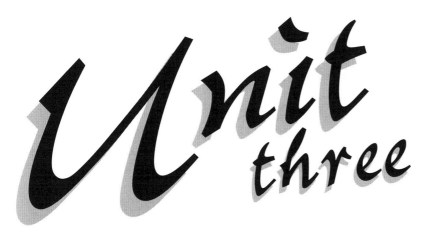

Understanding Personal Development

Introduction

In this unit you will learn about

- personal growth and development
- social and economic factors that can affect personal development
- self-concept
- major life changes and how people deal with them
- the types of support available.

This unit is assessed through an external assessment set by the awarding body with which your school or college is registered, and the grade you are given will be your grade for the unit. However, assessment evidence from your portfolio is still important, as it shows what you have learnt and how well you have understood the unit contents.

What you need to know	
1 Human growth and development	132
2 Social and economic factors affecting development	146
3 Self-concept	155
4 Life changes and types of support available to those experiencing major change	162

Unit 3.1
Human growth and development

You need to know the usual patterns by which people's bodies and minds develop from infancy to old age, and how most people become able to manage within society as they mature and develop an understanding of their emotions and relationships. You will be examining physical, intellectual, emotional, and social development. The following diagram illustrates the abilities that each of these types of development promotes in overall personal development.

EMOTIONAL to promote

confidence
a secure environment
ability to express feelings
ability to cope with anxieties
self–esteem

SOCIAL to promote

independence
awareness of others' needs
communication skills
anti–discriminatory attitudes
sense of social responsibility
comfort with own age group (peers)
good relations with adults
useful role models for others to follow
links between work/school and home
positive ideas about self

PERSONAL
DEVELOPMENT

INTELLECTUAL to promote

creativity
ability to listen
consideration of scientific ideas
observation
language
use of imagination
understanding numbers
enjoyment of art and music
learning through experience
concentration
reasoning

PHYSICAL to promote

bodily control
awareness of space
hand–eye coordination
manipulative skills

Physical development

The main stages in our physical development are growth, changes in puberty caused by hormones, maturity, and the ageing process.

Growth in the early stages of life

We develop most quickly during the first five years of life, during which the helpless baby grows into an independent, communicating, responsive child.

The physical skills which develop during infancy are called **motor skills** and depend upon accurate communication between the brain and the muscles. Therefore children who lack such communication will not reach the usual milestones at the same age as most children. However, all *comparative* stages are very general – some children reach them early, others late. Most tend to catch up given time. The following pictures show motor development comparative stages in the first years of an infant's life.

What do we mean by comparative stages?

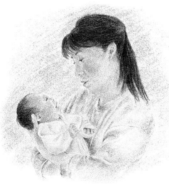

Newborn
Head flops back if unsupported.
Curls forward if put in sitting position.
Lies curled up if put on front.
If held with feet dangling onto a surface makes movements – the walk reflex.
Grasps anything which is put in hand – the grasp reflex.

unit three

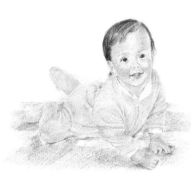

3 months
Begins to control head.
Back starting to straighten if held in sitting position.
Supports weight on bent arms if put on front.
If held upright, legs sag. Walking reflex is lost.
Plays with his or her fingers. Grasp reflex is lost.

6 months
Can raise head if lying on back.
Sits with hands on floor for support.
Supports weight on straight arms if put on front. Can roll over.
Can take weight on legs if held in standing position.
Can grasp objects nearby and pass to mouth and other hand.

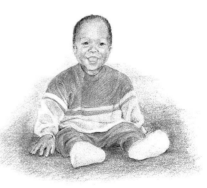

133

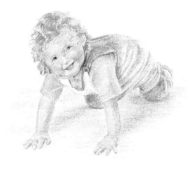

9 months
Has full control of head movements.
Can sit unsupported.
Can crawl clumsily.
Pulls up on furniture to standing and can 'walk' around furniture.
Can pick up small objects.

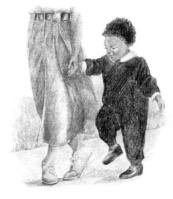

1 year
Can twist and stretch when sitting.
Crawls quickly.
Walks if hand is held to help balance.
Can throw a ball.

Physical development from 15 months to 5 years	
15 months	walks on own
18 months	walks backwards, climbs stairs
2 years	kicks a ball, draws
3 years	balances on one leg, dresses self
4 years	hops
5 years	skips

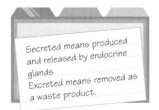

Secreted means produced and released by endocrine glands
Excreted means removed as a waste product.

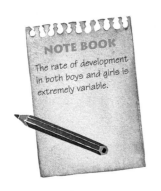

NOTE BOOK
The rate of development in both boys and girls is extremely variable.

Changes in puberty caused by hormones

Children usually continue growing steadily after the age of five until they reach adolescence, when growth slows down. It is regulated by messages from their **hormones**.

The hormones are secreted by glands known as **endocrine glands** and are circulated round the body in the blood stream. They are excreted by the kidneys in the urine when they are no longer needed (hence tests for the hormones that indicate pregnancy can be done through a urine test).

All hormone production is regulated by the **pituitary gland**, which is found at the base of the brain.

At **puberty** a great surge of hormonal activity causes boys and girls to develop into men and women capable of being sexually active. Children grow from infancy in a fairly accepting way, but at adolescence young people are able to be critical of their environment and themselves, and puberty can require quite painful adjustments to be made, especially as there are usually other outside pressures to cope with at the same time.

Puberty in boys occurs when hormones from the pituitary gland stimulate the secretion of male hormones. This causes

- a growth spurt in height
- strengthening of muscles
- more pronounced facial features
- thickening of the vocal cords and enlargement of the Adam's apple
- the voice to 'break'
- appearance of facial and body hair
- development of body odour

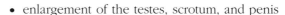

- enlargement of the testes, scrotum, and penis
- skin and hair to become more oily (acne may develop).

Changes begin internally at around 9 years old, although it is at least three years before any external signs develop. Puberty is generally completed by the age of 18.

Puberty in girls tends to begin and end earlier than in boys. It too depends on messages from the pituitary gland, stimulating the ovaries to secrete hormones. This begins about two years before menstruation.

Although as children girls are usually smaller than boys, their earlier puberty may mean that at the age of 13 they are on average about 2.5 cm (1 inch) taller than boys and that they finish their growth spurt before boys begin theirs. Changes at puberty include:

- an increase in height
- appearance of hair under the arms and in the pubic area
- broadening of the hips
- bodily fat being deposited in new places
- breast development
- **menstruation** (periods starting).

Maturity

Once through puberty, growth is complete and the body enters the third stage of its life cycle, that of **maturity**. During this period, men and women are able to have children, and bring them up to grow into adults themselves.

In humans this is the longest and most settled time of life, yet before it is over both men and women have to go through another process dictated by their hormone cycle. This is known as the **menopause.**

In women this is more dramatic than in men, and involves the pituitary ceasing to stimulate female hormone production so that menstruation ceases. One side-effect of this is that the bones may become brittle, leading to a condition called **osteoporosis**. Other symptoms may include sleeplessness, hot flushes, absent-mindedness, and irritability.

These last symptoms may also occur in men as their hormone balance shifts. Bear in mind that, around the age of 50, both men and women may be involved in external changes such as job shifts, and it is small wonder that this is often known as the 'mid-life crisis'.

The ageing process

The last stage of physical development is that of old age. Unlike puberty, it is not marked by dramatic changes, but is a gradual process of running down. Described on paper it looks very negative, but at the end of a lifetime of experiences, many people agree that

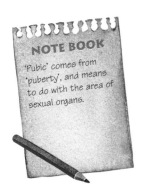

NOTE BOOK

'Pubic' comes from 'puberty', and means to do with the area of sexual organs.

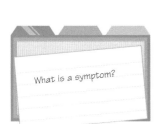

What is a symptom?

unit three

physical age is a case of mind over matter – if you don't mind, then it doesn't matter.

The rate of ageing and the extent of physical change involved vary widely between individuals. The following table describes the physical effects that ageing can produce.

Many of the changes occur as the body and its tissues actually shrink and the systems work less effectively.

Physical effects of ageing

1 Loss of colour in hair.

2 The eyes focus less well. Hearing may become impaired. Taste, smell, and touch are less acute. The sense of balance may become affected.

3 Weakened blood capillaries mean the skin bruises more easily and red patches may appear under the skin.

4 Breathing is less efficient as the lungs lose elasticity.

6 Arteries thicken inside, so blood circulates less freely. This reduces the oxygen supply and leads to sensitivity to the cold and a raised blood pressure.

7 The brain shrinks, affecting short-term memory. Nerves react more slowly, and responses are slower.

8 Skin loses its elasticity and forms sags and wrinkles.

9 Height loss as bones move closer together. Joints stiffen and enlarge. Muscles lose tone and size. Bones grow more brittle.

10 Digestive organs shrink, so meals need to be smaller.

11 The kidneys and bladder are less efficient.

An oral history project at a day care centre for the elderly involves people from three different stages of life.

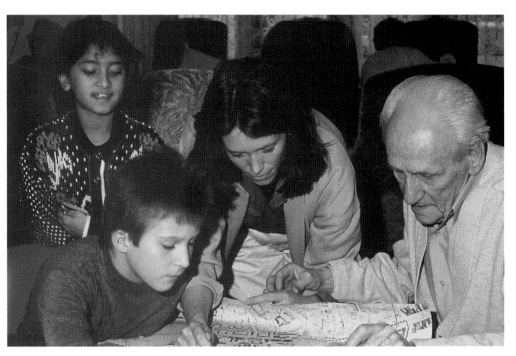

Intellectual development

There are three aspects of intellectual development to consider: cognition, language, and memory.

Cognition

The word 'cognition' is similar to 'recognition' and this tells us that it is to do with knowing and understanding.

The outline of cognitive development shown in the photographs below is a very simple representation, because so many outside influences affect children's growing understanding of the world.

Cognitive development
Bear in mind that people who have learning difficulties may not be able to complete a pattern of development such as the one shown here, although opportunity should always be offered to extend and stimulate, and it should never be assumed that development has ended.

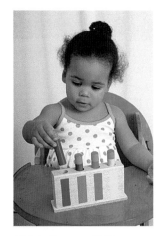

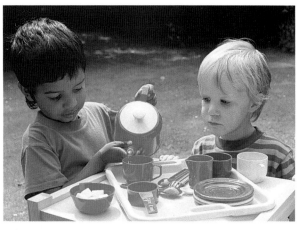

Birth to 2 years: child learns directly from his or her actions, rather than by thinking.

2–7 years: child lives only in the here and now. Only understands general ideas. Half lives in fantasy land.

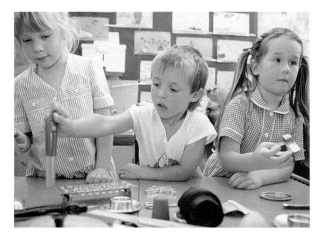

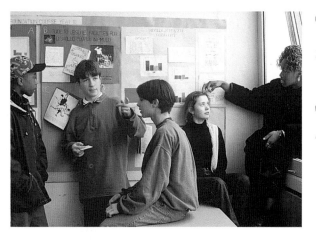

7–12 years: child can think logically about things which have been experienced.

12 years to adulthood: can reason about things without experiencing them.

It is tempting to analyse only how *children* learn. But we should not forget that all of us continue learning throughout our lives, in more or less the same way.

unit three

Language development

Development of language depends on effective learning. It takes practice – listening, speaking, responding. Babies speak in 'scribble' talk. Then, as they develop, they become more skilled at forming words. The number of words we know increases as we talk and listen and read throughout life. Language is a tool we can use to achieve clear thought and good communication. All learners – children, young and old, able-bodied and disabled – need time, patience, and clear sounds to copy so that as many words as possible can be remembered and used properly.

Language is a key to empowerment for all people, including those with no speech, those with hearing impairment, and those who learn slowly.

Infants soon respond to their names and those of their family and toys, and smile when they say these names. They babble to themselves and talk to things as well as people.

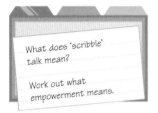

What does 'scribble' talk mean?

Work out what empowerment means.

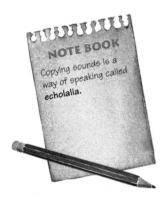

NOTE BOOK
Copying sounds is a way of speaking called **echolalia**.

ACTIVITY A

1 Write down ten things you learnt before you were five.

2 Then write down ten things you have learnt during the last six months.

3 Against each thing that you have written down, write how you learnt it, from the following list:

- enthusiasm
- copying
- making mistakes
- encouragement
- practice
- you wanted to improve
- praise
- useful feedback on progress
- having ideas
- success being necessary
- from a book
- one thing leading to another
- guessing

4 Are the learning methods different for the two lists in 1 and 2? If so, why could this be?

5 Record your conclusions in an appropriate and imaginative way.

◀▶ Extension opportunity

Link your conclusions to the four stages of your own cognitive development, as outlined in the photographs on page 137.

Memory

When you begin looking after others, you may find that some don't always remember what you tell or show them.

Children learn to remember things for longer as they grow older and are encouraged to repeat sounds and experiences. Later they respond to pictures and then to letters and words.

People with mental health problems make wrong connections with the clues the world gives to them. They may not recognise objects for what they are, but instead may see them as threatening or harmful. No amount of reasoning will convince them that they are misinterpreting what they see, and they are not able to remember previous experiences in a helpful way.

As we grow older, there is more to forget, so our memories seem to suffer. When we are stressed, our concentration slips and we make mistakes. Old people may find it easier to remember their childhood than what happened last week.

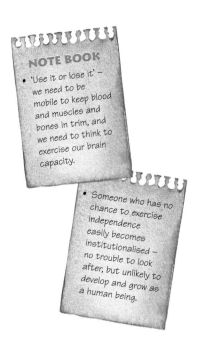

NOTE BOOK

- 'Use it or lose it' – we need to be mobile to keep blood and muscles and bones in trim, and we need to think to exercise our brain capacity.

- Someone who has no chance to exercise independence easily becomes institutionalised – no trouble to look after, but unlikely to develop and grow as a human being.

Emotional development

Good emotional development is encouraged by bonding with others and developing independence and self-confidence.

Bonding

Sound emotional development depends on an individual forming close affection for other people. In infancy this is known as bonding, and begins when a baby is cuddled closely. This means that the main carer is involved, usually the mother, before the circle of affection expands.

When people have learning difficulties, this simple form of bonding may extend beyond childhood. With others, it grows into love and liking for others. When bonding does not occur within the early weeks of life, children can grow up finding it difficult to give or receive affection.

The signs of bonding extend into adult life, and include wanting to touch each other, long eye contact, and response to voice.

Independence

If a person is secure in a loving framework, independence can develop. It begins slowly, in the same way as walking skills do, with practice, encouragement, and approval. Small children dare to venture away from their parents until as adolescents they are truly separate people, held to the family only by the invisible links forged during infancy.

All carers should aim to allow those they work with to remain themselves, involved as much as possible in their own care. Independence is also examined in Unit One (page 68).

unit three

The balance of independence

INDEPENDENCE
• walking alone
• managing money
• making choices
• looking after oneself
• going one's own pace
• using all available help and aids to enable home living

RISK
• falling
• getting into debt
• making mistakes
• not maintaining good health
• taking a long time
• isolation from the community

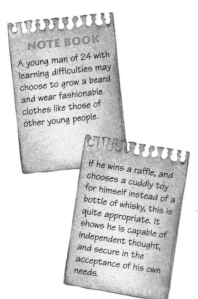

NOTE BOOK

A young man of 24 with learning difficulties may choose to grow a beard and wear fashionable clothes like those of other young people.

If he wins a raffle, and chooses a cuddly toy for himself instead of a bottle of whisky, this is quite appropriate. It shows he is capable of independent thought, and secure in the acceptance of his own needs.

Do you know the meaning of celibate, heterosexual and homosexual, and deviance?

Emotional security and social ease

A basic human need is to be loved and valued. It is normal for everyone to feel unwanted at some time, but some people feel like this most of the time. The feeling can demonstrate itself in many ways, such as by unacceptable behaviour, withdrawal, or seeking attention. Reacting in those ways is often easier for the individual than discussing the matter openly, either because they feel reluctant to express their feelings or because they have no language to describe how they feel.

Those who do not live in a family group may well gain their emotional security from their friends and workmates. People of the same age or status as each other are called **peers**. It is inappropriate for children of four, for example, to feel comfortable only in the company of people of their grandparents' age. They need to be able to get on with other young children.

People with disabilities need to have the chance to mix with able-bodied friends. This process is called **normalisation**, which means giving everybody access to different styles of living so that they can exercise choice about their lifestyle to the best of their ability.

Personal sexuality is a source of anxiety to some. It is not only concerned with love and acceptance, but also with basic human instincts that can be hard to control. Some people need help in handling sexual urges, and education about the need for responsibility and discretion.

There is the same variety of sexuality among clients as there is among carers. Both groups will include those who choose to remain celibate, both heterosexual and homosexual people, and those who have sexual deviances which are not generally accepted in society.

Adolescence, maturity, mid-life, and old age all bring concerns about sexuality which may need to be confronted and resolved. Sexual counselling is a refined skill, and specialist practitioners should be recommended when the need arises.

Self-confidence

With successful independence comes self-confidence, although it is normal for everyone to feel shy and unsure at times, however old or mature they may appear to be. But self-confidence is unattainable without a sound basis of love and security laid down in childhood.

Social development

Co-operation and relationships

The pictures on this page illustrate the pattern of social development in children between 6 months old and 7 years old.

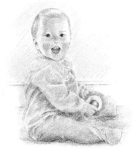

***6 months**: smiles, attracts attention, makes noises*

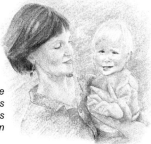

***9 months**: sees those outside the family as strangers and needs reassuring often*

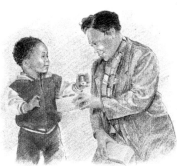

***1 year**: begins to do as he or she is told, begins to 'help'*

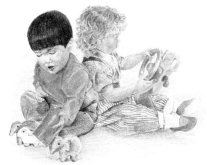

***2 years**: plays in a group of children, but very selfishly*

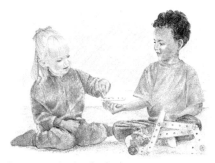

***3 years**: understands sharing*

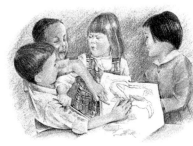

***4 years**: needs the company of other children but may quarrel with them frequently*

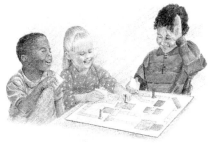

***5–7 years**: plays co-operatively and understands that rules are necessary*

unit three

Babies are at first completely self-centred. Gradually they begin to realise that other people exist, and so their social development begins. The family is the first group of people of which children become aware, but still they think first of themselves. Then they begin to test the family, in order to discover the limits of the boundaries of their expected behaviour.

Social development is shown by the progressive stages in which children play, and this may be reflected in the way that adults react when they join groups with which they are not familiar:

- solitary play – playing alone
- parallel play – playing next to others but not communicating
- looking-on play – watching without joining in
- joining-in play – doing the same thing as everyone else
- co-operative play – belonging to the group and sharing activities.

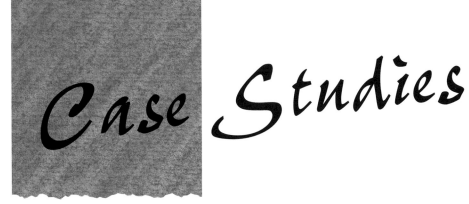

Case Studies

Case study 1.1   Hill Hall

Ann is beginning to come to grips with the emotional stress of working with disabled children, and Molly is keen that she doesn't lose touch with the reality of the average child's development. She asks Ann to do a comparative study of Usha, a Hindu girl with physical and mental disabilities resulting from cerebral palsy, and Ann's sister Lucy, who is the same age and has no disabilities. Ann is to begin by writing down the main characteristics of development in the different stages of life, starting with infancy and ending with old age.

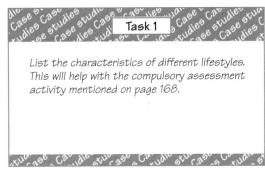

Task 1

List the characteristics of different lifestyles. This will help with the compulsory assessment activity mentioned on page 168.

Case study 1.2   Netherfield Community Care

Sometimes members of the Polish community have visitors from their homeland. Often their grandchildren are brought to see them. As Christmas draws near, Mikhail asks Debbie to help him to arrange some activities for these children over the holiday period.

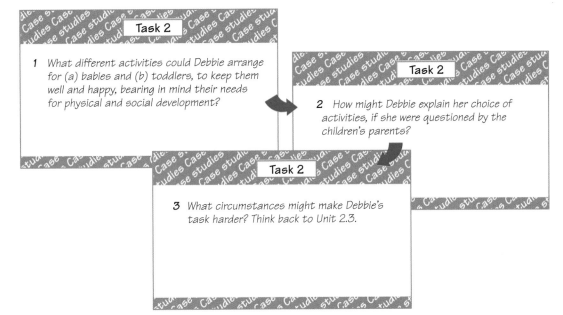

Task 2

1   What different activities could Debbie arrange for (a) babies and (b) toddlers, to keep them well and happy, bearing in mind their needs for physical and social development?

Task 2

2   How might Debbie explain her choice of activities, if she were questioned by the children's parents?

Task 2

3   What circumstances might make Debbie's task harder? Think back to Unit 2.3.

unit three case studies

Case study 1.3   Down Way School and The Thatched Cottage

Mark and Jalwinder meet Ann, who is excited because she has gained a high grade for her study about Usha and Lucy. They decide to work together to compare Tim's development with Rosa's.

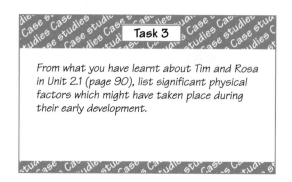

Task 3

From what you have learnt about Tim and Rosa in Unit 2.1 (page 90), list significant physical factors which might have taken place during their early development.

Multiple Choice Questions

1.1 The menopause is the name given to physical changes which take place in

  a infancy

  b old age

  c adulthood

  d adolescence

1.2 Which of the following life stages comes after puberty?

  a old age

  b infancy

  c maturity

  d childhood

1.3 Intellectual development involves

  a memory

  b motor skills

  c osteoporosis

  d bonding

1.4 Which of the following is a direct result of independence?

  a language development

  b stereotyping

  c self-confidence

  d menopause

1.5 Changes at puberty are caused by

  a diet

  b ageing

  c hormones

  d gender

1.6 When a mother and baby forge strong emotional links, this is known as

  a motherhood

  b recognition

  c bonding

  d contact

Note: These questions are for you to test your knowledge. There is no formal multiple choice test in this GNVQ.

unit three

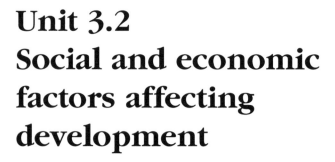

Unit 3.2
Social and economic factors affecting development

Social and economic factors have an impact on an individual's development. The social factors to consider are culture, gender, access to services including education, family, friends, housing and environment, and ethnicity. These are considered together in the following section. Isolation, discrimination, and stereotyping are then covered separately.

Social factors affecting development

Health inequalities

With death rates in Europe being at the lowest point in the history of human society, and infectious diseases having declined dramatically, inequalities in health ought to have disappeared. But, in fact, socio-economic factors continue to have an effect on whether or not communities thrive.

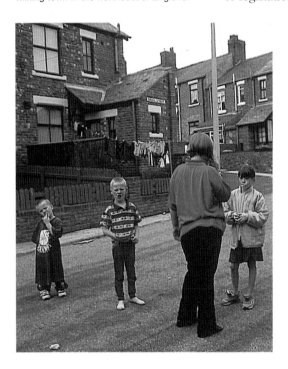

Children play in the street in a former mining town in the northeast of England.

The desire for environmental health has given rise to a framework of legislation throughout Europe. In a bid to improve water and air quality and to limit noise pollution, housing and building regulations have been drawn up and **Health and Safety at Work** (HASAW) legislation has been passed. This is not the case in less well-developed parts of the world, where social differences are more marked than they are in the United Kingdom, although the World Health Organisation (WHO) has drawn attention to the direct relationship between the health of a population and a pure water supply.

Yet, despite this, health inequalities still exist. Everyone has the same needs to enable them to grow and develop to their full potential, but because society is made up of such a complex mix of people, some are able to enjoy better health than others. Social deprivation may exist in western society masked by apparent affluence. There is a complex inter-relation between the health of the people in a nation and their housing, nutrition, occupation, education, and financial resources.

Social attitudes, modes of life, cultural customs, and individual beliefs may support healthy living or, alternatively, contribute to ill health.

The role of the family in the development of individuals

Families, in their raising of children, play a crucial role in the development of individuals. We carry all through our lives the good and the bad things we learnt from our families in childhood.

A family is a group of people of various ages, related by birth, marriage, or adoption. It is the basic unit of society.

Society is built up of families

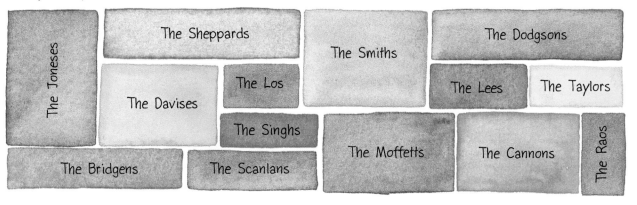

In a wider context the family unit could be a father, his children, and his girlfriend, or a mother and daughter and her boyfriend, or a couple in a caring loving homosexual relationship who live together.

The three roles of **protection**, **provision**, and **support** (see the table below) are most intense when there are children in the family, but they combine throughout family members' lives. Some close families protect, provide for, and support many members very actively over periods of time. Other families move apart and the roles are then

The role of the family

PROTECTION	PROVISION	SUPPORT
• food • shelter • warmth • clothing • training in how to be social individuals • immunisation against disease • providing experiences to increase independence	• protection (see previous list) • education • financial help • support (see following list) • role models • advice on problems	• love and affection • understanding • mutual respect • sense of belonging • promoting self-esteem • encouraging independence • helping one another as circumstances change • visiting and companionship • maintaining family traditions to give a sense of continuity

unit three

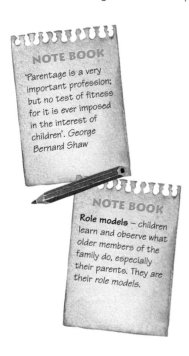

taken over by friends or society. Much depends on learnt family behaviour patterns, circumstances, personalities, and cultural expectations.

Children from families where protection, provision, and support are absent or incomplete, or parenting is inadequate – in particular when love and affection are missing – do not thrive emotionally or physically and are said to be **deprived**. Such children may grow into adults who have difficulty in forming satisfactory relationships, as they have been unable to develop fully as individuals.

Family life and divorce

- In 1998, around 1 in 4 children affected by divorce were under 5 years old, and about 7 in 10 were aged under 10 years old.

- Almost 1 in 4 children born in 1979 was likely to have been affected by divorce before the age of 16.

- The younger people are when they enter the first relationship in which they live with their partner, the less likely they are to marry that partner.

- In 1972, 7% of children lived in lone-parent families. By 1999 this had increased to 23%.

- In 1998–99, over half of men aged 20–24 lived with their parents, and just over a third of all women of the same age.

- In 1996–97, stepfamilies with dependent children accounted for 8% of all families with dependent children in Great Britain.

- State benefits are targeted on the lower earning groups.

- Until they are 18, it is difficult for young people to claim from social security.

Changes in relationship formation have meant that living arrangements and family structures have become more diverse than at the start of the 1990s. Nevertheless, families continue to play a very important role in people's lives, with family contact and support being common.

ACTIVITY A

Think about
- a single father caring for two children under five years old

- a teenager who has left home because of emotional abuse

- a baby found in a telephone kiosk

- an elderly widower with advanced Parkinson's disease, living alone.

Make a list of their physical, social, intellectual, and emotional needs.

Will these be different from the needs of similar individuals in a stable family situation?

Will it be possible for the people's needs to be met, in their current lifestyles?

Discuss your findings in a group.

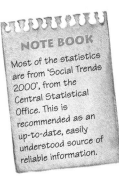

NOTE BOOK

Most of the statistics are from 'Social Trends 2000', from the Central Statistical Office. This is recommended as an up-to-date, easily understood source of reliable information.

Homelessness

- In 1998–99, a quarter of all households accepted as being homeless in England were in that situation because parents, relatives, or friends were no longer willing or able to accommodate them, especially young homeless people.

- Older homeless people identified family crises, such as widowhood or marriage breakdown, alongside eviction, redundancy, and mental illness, as reasons for homelessness.

- In 1998–99, local authorities in England made a total of 245,480 decisions on applications for housing for homeless households. Of these, more than 105,470 were deemed eligible for assistance.

- In 1996–97, about 14% of households in England lived in 'poor housing' – unfit, needing substantial repair, or requiring essential modernisation. Most such accommodation had private tenants.

How social factors influence lifestyle choices

Culture, family, friends, housing and environment, and ethnicity are all social factors affecting people's development. We have seen that families form societies, and, as individuals often choose their friends from similar backgrounds living nearby, so cultural and behavioural patterns are repeated. These can influence lifestyle choices (see page 107) such as child-rearing patterns, smoking, alcohol and substance abuse, dietary habits, exercise levels, attitudes to preventive health care, etc. Individuals' choices are also affected by their physical and mental qualities, their personal styles and dispositions, and class reinforcement of lifestyle. Community health services are attempting to iron out inequalities by ensuring access to services and education, with far-reaching results in some ethnic-minority groups.

Women are more inclined than men to take care of their health. This is accounted for by differences in behaviour, such as women being less likely than men to be involved in hazardous occupations and women having different attitudes to smoking and alcohol consumption. The differences are becoming less marked as men's life expectancy is raised and behaviour boundaries are less defined.

Isolation, discrimination, and stereotyping

Sometimes individuals become separated from society and are then said to be **isolated**. This means that they are unable to interact normally with others. It might happen because of personality, mental or physical illness, or mobility or communication problems. Extremes of poverty or richness also tend to isolate individuals, as does any factor far removed from what is considered normal in society. People who are isolated are denied the right to personal development, and carers need to be aware of this so that they can take steps to correct any tendency to isolation in their clients. (See page 104 on responses to stress.)

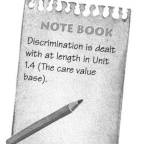

NOTE BOOK

Discrimination is dealt with at length in Unit 1.4 (The care value base).

unit three

ACTIVITY B

1 Find an advertisement showing a stereotyped individual, group, or situation.

2 Describe it as the advertiser wishes you to see it.

3 Imagine what might be the reality behind the stereotype.

4 Think of the disadvantages which might follow the portrayal of an ideal rather than a real image, as far as the reader is concerned.

5 Draw some speech bubbles coming out of the mouths of those in the picture contradicting the image presented in the illustration.

C2.2

6 Use the activity to produce a page suitable for inclusion in a student leaflet designed to raise awareness of discriminatory behaviour. Use a computer if you wish.

IT2.3

How stereotyping individuals and groups can lead to discriminatory behaviour

When we **stereotype** a person or a group, we stop seeing them as individuals and mass them together under a single label which robs them of personality. Using stereotypes is a lazy way of thinking – it saves the trouble of finding out more about people.

Stereotyping begins with making assumptions, which may be based on our first impressions:

- use of language
- accent
- area the person lives in
- education
- clothes
- car/house ownership
- occupation.

All these and more affect the way we first feel about people. If we do not get to know them better they may remain fixed in our minds as stereotypes.

Advertisements, magazines, and television all feed stereotypes. Drama often portrays people as shallow images with no past or future. Advertisements depict ideal situations with no problems or personal hardships. Magazines show rose-tinted, unattainable situations, which the average person cannot hope to achieve.

When we see people as 'cardboard cut-outs', with no blood in their veins, feelings in their minds, or personal histories, dreams, or disappointments, we are stereotyping them. By denying them an existence as individuals, we cease to have sympathy for them and the seeds of discrimination are sown.

Economic factors affecting development

Poverty leaves some people unable to share the amenities or facilities provided within an affluent society. This means that they may not be able to do what they would like to in their neighbourhood. They may not be able to carry out occupational obligations because of limited resources. For example, a low income might make it difficult for a person to afford to travel to work, or to buy special clothing needed at work. People who are poor may also be disadvantaged as a result of illness or accident, or lack of factors positively influencing their good health.

A person's or a family's income decides what money there is to spend on life's essentials – food, clothing, housing – and what money is to spare for things that are enjoyable yet not strictly speaking necessary, such as holidays, magazines, videos, make-up. People on relatively low incomes remain relatively disadvantaged with regard to early retirement, unemployment, and redundancy, while single-parent status, disablement, and the rise in the elderly population can all contribute to the rise in poverty today.

unit three

Self-esteem

People with high self-esteem

- have a realistic view of their abilities, even if they are few
- have confidence
- are not worried by criticism
- enjoy well-being
- join in willingly
- make friends easily
- succeed
- are independent

People with low self-esteem

- underestimate what they can do
- are inward-looking and unconfident
- are sensitive to criticism
- get depressed easily
- join in reluctantly
- find it hard to make friends
- underachieve
- find independence difficult

Low incomes affect health, employment prospects, and education, while all negative social and economic factors have a bad effect on personal self-esteem.

Building self-esteem

Self-esteem means how you value yourself. Confident people feel good about themselves and have high self-esteem. People who see themselves as having no value have low self-esteem. The table on the left compares the attributes of people with high and low self-esteem.

Self-esteem matters for carers as well as clients. Its foundations are laid in childhood, so carers working with children need to be aware of its importance.

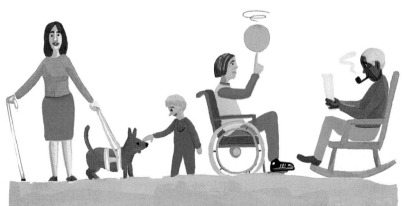

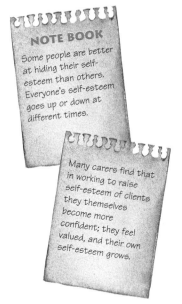

NOTE BOOK

Some people are better at hiding their self-esteem than others. Everyone's self-esteem goes up or down at different times.

Many carers find that in working to raise self-esteem of clients they themselves become more confident; they feel valued, and their own self-esteem grows.

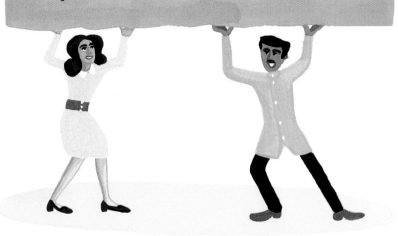

Clients' self-esteem is raised by
- praise
- encouragement
- the chance to make decisions
- being listened to
- independence
- feeling valued
- the chance to succeed
- belonging to a group
- having responsibility
- having even small efforts acknowledged

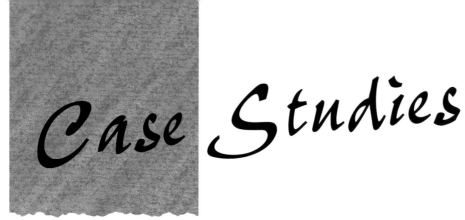

Case Studies

Case study 2.1 Netherfield Community Care

You met Mishka in the case studies in Unit Two (see page 90). Her son with schizophrenia is called Jan. His medication has been successfully changed, and his condition is much more stable, but he finds making friends difficult.

Task 1

1 If Jan lived in your neighbourhood, how might he be helped to meet other people?

2 What is the danger of his spending too much time alone?

Case study 2.2 Down Way School and The Thatched Cottage

(Continued from Unit 3.1, page 144)

Task 2

1 What are the principal social factors currently affecting Tim and Rosa?

2 How can the workplaces help to minimise any adverse effects of these social factors?

Case study 2.3   Hill Hall

One of the main aims of the staff at Hill Hall is to give their clients as rich a social life as is possible within the confines of their disabilities. Ann brings into work a list of the social and economic factors affecting development, and decides to work out how they may have affected her clients.

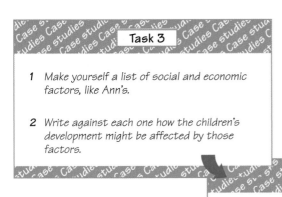

Task 3

1   Make yourself a list of social and economic factors, like Ann's.

2   Write against each one how the children's development might be affected by those factors.

Task 3

3   How might Hill Hall staff minimise any negative effects created by the children's learning difficulties?

Multiple Choice Questions

2.1 Poverty can give rise to

    a immunisation

    b environmental factors

    c physical development

    d health inequalities

2.2 When an individual becomes withdrawn from other people it is called

    a isolation

    b ethnicity

    c identity

    d discrimination

2.3 Which of the following is an economic factor affecting development?

    a culture

    b gender

    c income

    d age

2.4 Which of the following is NOT a social factor affecting personal development?

    a infancy

    b family

    c friends

    d discrimination

Note: These questions are for you to test your knowledge. There is no formal multiple choice test in this GNVQ.

Unit 3.3
Self-concept

We all have an idea of who we really are, how we would like to appear to the outside world, and what we would change if we could. It is important to understand the reasons for this opinion of ourselves.

Self-concept means the way in which we see ourselves, and it is very much affected by how other people see us. We view ourselves in the mirror of other people's opinions, and the reflection we see depends on many aspects of our background, experience, and personality. Factors influencing self-concept include:

- education
- gender
- emotional maturity
- sexual maturity
- appearance
- age
- culture
- relationships
- work.

Education

Education is not to be confused with intellectual development. It is to do with our upbringing and our schooling, and how much this has done to enrich our self-confidence and self-esteem.

unit three

ACTIVITY A

1 Think about the following statements:

a Feminism has ceased to be a new phenomenon in the United Kingdom and some maintain that women have overtaken men in matters of gender equality.

b As single mothers bring up children successfully, some of those children may begin to question the need for constant fathering.

c Male unemployed graduates outnumber female unemployed graduates.

d Females begin to be better qualified than men. However, more men than women hold the most powerful jobs.

2 Working in a small group, decide some possible results of the four situations 1 a-d and how they might affect individuals during their

a infancy and childhood

b adolescence

c early adulthood

d mid-life

e old age.

3 Share your group's opinions with your tutor group, and record those that the majority considers to be significant.

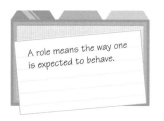

A role means the way one is expected to behave.

Gender

Gender means sex; male or female. All around us there are images of how men and women are supposed to behave. These images are stereotypes, and they can be very unhelpful to an individual trying to establish their own identity. Traditionally women were stereotyped as housewives, and men as money earners, but these roles are no longer relevant to many people's lives.

This is an important factor in an individual's self-concept; without confidence in your gender role it is hard to know quite who you are, and our perception of ourselves can depend to a large extent on what we think is other people's opinion of us.

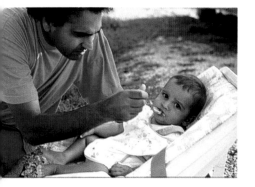

Emotional maturity

We all need to love and be loved. Without the bonding experience described earlier (page 139), it is difficult for adults to form the normal, accepting friendships which indicate emotional maturity. Those with low self-esteem find it hard to see anything reflected off those around them which shows there to be anything lovable in themselves.

In our society, which promotes the image of the ideal body, it can be especially easy for people who have disfigurements or deformities to see themselves as ugly. If, during their education and upbringing, they are constantly respected as individuals worthy of receiving love, they are more likely to develop into emotionally mature adults.

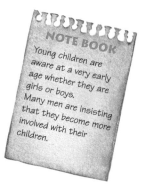

NOTE BOOK

Young children are aware at a very early age whether they are girls or boys.
Many men are insisting that they become more involved with their children.

Conversely, some adults who are emotionally immature feel themselves to be ugly when they are not. This is quite common during growing up. Most people grow out of it as they see themselves to be accepted as normal people by their friends.

Sexual maturity

After puberty, a person is sexually mature. It is a physical state brought about, as we have seen, by hormonal changes. During the process many emotional changes also take place, and a person's self-concept often becomes confused, but this is usually only temporary. With sexual maturity comes the ability to be sexually active. If emotional maturity lags behind, this can result in sexual behaviour which is promiscuous or inappropriate.

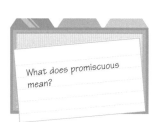

What does promiscuous mean?

People with learning difficulties may be sexually mature, yet not have the social or emotional maturity to know when, where, or how it is acceptable to have sexual relationships. People with psychiatric illnesses may be unable to control their sexual urges, despite being sexually mature.

These complications make sexual maturity a complex factor in a person's self-concept.

Appearance

We have examined how we 'see' ourselves and how we may think others 'see' us, but have been thinking about ideas rather than what is simply seen with the eyes. Now we come to actual appearance; physical characteristics, clothing, and body language. We all have confused images when we think of our physical characteristics, when all most people see is a perfectly normal person.

So we cover our confusion with clothes, either different from everyone else's if we want to make a point, or as like everyone else's as possible if we want people to associate us with a particular group.

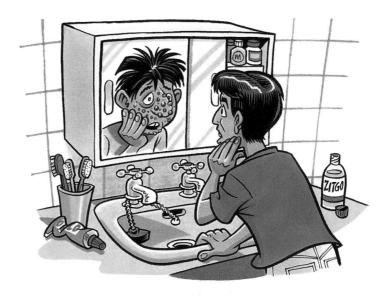

ACTIVITY B

1 What image might the people in the photographs on the right be hoping to project to those who see them?

2 Are they trying to be different from or the same as others in their group?

3 Conduct two surveys among a cross-section of males and females to see which clothes they prefer to wear.

---

a
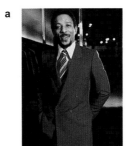

b
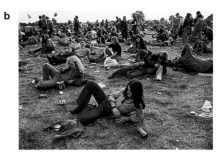

c
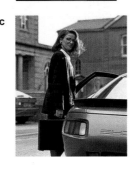

d
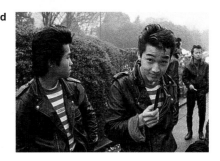

Age

Society expects people to behave in certain ways according to their age. Use the following activity to help you think about this.

ACTIVITY C

1 Describe how you think

a a 7-year-old girl,

b a 30-year-old woman,

c an 18-year-old man, and

d a 70-year-old woman

would behave

- in a queue at the fish and chip shop
- on a bus
- caught in a rain storm.

2 If, instead, they behaved in another, very unpredictable way, talk about what this might suggest about how they think of themselves and their age.

Culture

Our ideas of ourselves are formed by the people who surround us.

'Little girls should be seen and not heard'

'Little boys don't cry'

'Men must work and women must weep'

Sayings like this give us ideals, and when we break away from them we sometimes become stronger in our self-concept and sometimes feel guilty because we have not done what is expected of us.

Different cultures impose different expectations of language, music, literature, religion, and lifestyle. Sometimes men are very dominant, and women are subservient – culture and gender combining as factors affecting self-image.

Some examples of cultural expectations are arranged marriages, 'suitable' employment, respect for grandparents. The response of our culture to our chosen lifestyle is an important factor in how we feel about ourselves as adults.

Relationships

As we grow up and become independent, our relationships extend beyond the family. We often adjust our behaviour according to the company we are in, to try to gain approval. Our conduct changes subtly as our self-concept shifts when we see ourselves through others' eyes.

ACTIVITY D

1 List the people you have met today.

2 Describe your relationship with each of them. Here are some relationships which may fit:
admirer, friend, acquaintance, colleague, sister/brother, member of the public, employee, son/daughter, student, stranger.

3 Describe how your behaviour has changed as you have responded to each person.

Whom do we admire?

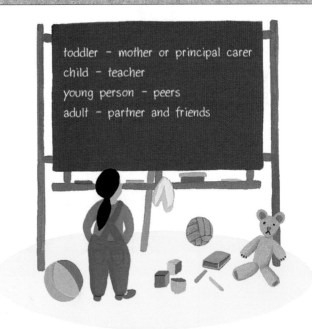

> toddler – mother or principal carer
> child – teacher
> young person – peers
> adult – partner and friends

Work

'What do you do?' is often the first question you are asked after your name. Many people see themselves mainly in the light of their jobs and when answering, we say: 'I *am* a nurse', 'I *am* a footballer', 'I *am* a classroom assistant', not 'I *work as* a nurse', 'I *work as* a footballer', 'I *work as* a classroom assistant' – which shows how much we identify with our jobs. This is a problem when people become unemployed, stay at home to care for someone else, or retire, after seeing their work as an essential part of their existence.

For people who have never worked, and who may have had many rejections during their search for work, self-esteem can be very low. It is important for the community to reinforce that everybody is precious and important, regardless of their employed status.

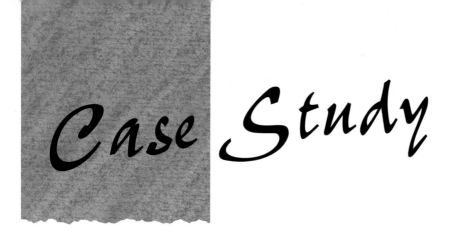

Case Study

Case study 3.1   Hill Hall

(continuing Ann's work on Usha and Lucy, case study 1.1, page 143)

Molly asks Ann to identify the factors that influence an individual's self-concept, keeping it general and not specific to either Usha or Lucy.

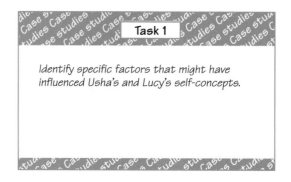

Task 1

Identify specific factors that might have influenced Usha's and Lucy's self-concepts.

Multiple Choice Questions

3.1 Education, appearance, maturity, and relationships all affect an individual's

  a *self-destruction*

  b *selfishness*

  c *self-analysis*

  d *self-concept*

3.2 Self-concept means

  a *the way in which we see ourselves*

  b *other people's opinion of us*

  c *that we fit into society easily*

  d *that we are self-educated*

3.3 Sexual maturity occurs after

  a *relationships*

  b *independence*

  c *puberty*

  d *education*

3.4 Which of the following form part of a person's culture?

  a *age and gender*

  b *adolescence and intellect*

  c *self-confidence and health*

  d *language and religion*

Note: These questions are for you to test your knowledge. There is no formal multiple choice test in this GNVQ.

unit three

Unit 3.4
Life changes and types of support available to those experiencing major change

No two people respond to change in the same way. Our personalities, upbringing, and experience all combine to give us a particular view of ourselves, which in turn colours the way in which we cope with life's ups and downs.

Sometimes the things that happen to people are expected and sometimes they are a surprise – either enjoyable or unpleasant. Either way, people can react in a variety of ways which you need to know about if you are to respond sympathetically to those you look after, or to understand the effects of life experiences on yourself.

The things that happen to us fall into two main groups; those we expect, which are **predictable**, and those we do not, which are **unpredictable**.

Predictable events

The predictable events in a person's life might include:

- starting school
- starting work
- leaving home
- marriage
- having children
- changing job
- moving home
- retirement.

It is easy to think that these are positive experiences, leading to new possibilities, yet even exciting events cause stress in our lives, especially when we worry that things may not turn out well.

Activity A asks you to think about your feelings when some predictable events happened to you. What you felt is shared by everyone confronted by **change**, from a small child starting play-school to a mature adult changing a job, a patient recovering from an operation and about to go home, or a young person with a disability getting a first car, which will bring independence and mobility.

ACTIVITY A

1 Think of some predictable events that have happened to you.

2 What did you feel as they came nearer?

Here is a list to help:

apprehension, uncertainty, loneliness, anxiety, inadequacy, fear of failure, fear of the known, sick, fear of responsibility, fear of looking foolish, nervous, tension, excitement.

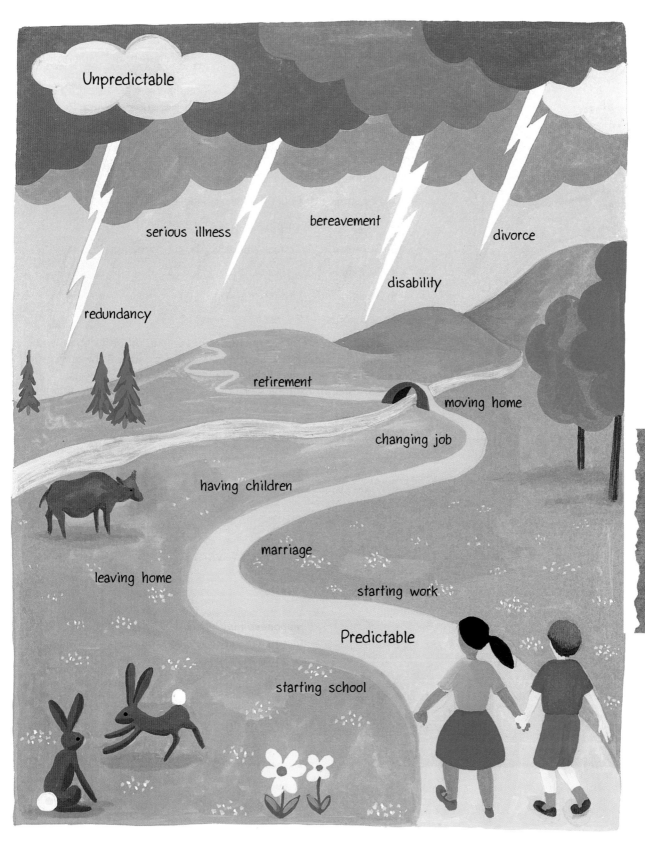

Unpredictable events

The unpredictable events in people's lives often bring *elements of bereavement*, which means **loss**. The loss may be in the form of redundancy, where a job is lost; serious illness, where health is lost; disability, where ability is lost; divorce or separation, where a relationship is lost; and bereavement, where a person's physical presence is lost through death.

The stages of bereavement have been mapped, and apply broadly to all the unpredictable events listed:

1 Denial and disbelief – 'I don't believe it'.

2 Anger – 'How can this happen to me?'

3 Depression – 'Things will never be the same again'.

4 Despair – 'I can't go on'.

5 Adjustment – 'Life must go on'.

6 Acceptance – 'It's up to me now'.

Individuals react to these unexpected events in different ways, some adjusting more quickly than others. Much depends on the amount of additional stress in their lives at the same time, their personality, and their self-esteem. Examples of possible responses to predictable and unpredictable events are given in the diagram below.

Possible responses to events

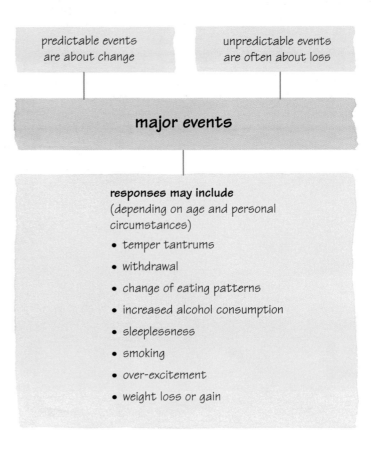

predictable events
are about change

unpredictable events
are often about loss

major events

responses may include
(depending on age and personal circumstances)

- temper tantrums
- withdrawal
- change of eating patterns
- increased alcohol consumption
- sleeplessness
- smoking
- over-excitement
- weight loss or gain

Types of support available to those experiencing major change

When important changes occur in life, individuals seek comfort and help in many ways.

Family support

People look for support in the way which is best for themselves and for the situation they find themselves in. Many turn to their families first.

Social support

Social support can come from friends, colleagues, and the community in which we live:

- religious leaders
- clubs and social groups
- school or college
- ethnic community groups.

Professional help

Professional help can be general, or specific for certain situations. For example, **medical help** could come from the family doctor, practice nurse, special clinic, pharmacist, community nurse or health visitor, or health centre; **financial help** could come from social security benefits, local authorities, or educational grants.

Some people need convincing that welfare benefits are their right – elderly people sometimes view them as charity. Since in this country we all pay tax either through work or on the things that we buy, everyone in need is entitled to state benefits. They are preferable to private loans and credit schemes (hire purchase) which may grow beyond the borrower's control. **Advisory help** includes

- public services (e.g. Citizens' Advice Bureau)
- voluntary organisations with specialist knowledge (e.g. British Red Cross Society, Diabetic Association, Mencap, National Society for Prevention of Cruelty to Children, Alcoholics Anonymous, The Terence Higgins Trust)
- counselling services.

ACTIVITY B

1 Read again your list of predictable major events and your reactions to them (see Activity A, page 162).

2 Remind yourself how you were helped to cope with your feelings until you felt able to manage alone.

3 Sort them under the following headings: family help, social help, professional help.

4 Record the information in a suitable way.

unit three

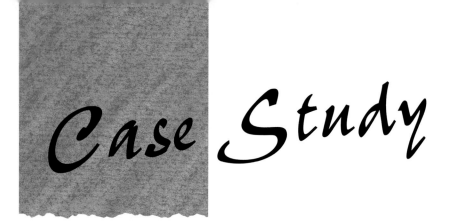

Case Study

Case study 4.1   The Thatched Cottage, Netherfield Community Care, and Down Way School

(looking back on the stories of Rosa, Mishka, and Tim in Unit 2.1, pages 90-91)

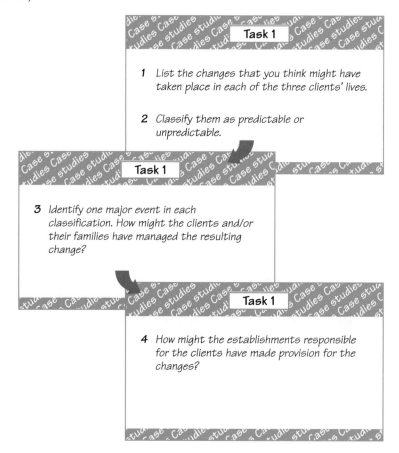

Task 1

1   List the changes that you think might have taken place in each of the three clients' lives.

2   Classify them as predictable or unpredictable.

Task 1

3   Identify one major event in each classification. How might the clients and/or their families have managed the resulting change?

Task 1

4   How might the establishments responsible for the clients have made provision for the changes?

Multiple Choice Questions

4.1 Which of the following is a *predictable* major life event?

a *disability*

b *having children*

c *divorce*

d *illness*

4.2 If the main earner in the family is made redundant, which one of the following would be the *most* useful?

a *counselling by Relate*

b *consultation with the family's GP*

c *professional help from social services*

d *appointment of an advocate*

4.3 Which of the following phrases *best* describes the impact on a family of the birth of a child with severe physical disabilities?

a *an acquired disability problem*

b *problems with intellectual development*

c *a factor influencing self-concept*

d *an unpredictable major event in life*

4.4 When someone goes through a major life change, social support may come from

a *an ethnic community group*

b *Citizens' Advice Bureau*

c *a pharmacist*

d *Mencap*

Note: These questions are for you to test your knowledge. There is no formal multiple choice test in this GNVQ.

unit three

Compulsory Assessment Activity

Assessment of Unit Three

As stated on page 5, this unit is assessed differently from Units One and Two. Assessment is carried out by the awarding body with which you are registered, through what is called a **controlled assignment**. The optional tasks and activities described throughout the unit chapter (pages 131-167) have been designed to make it easier for you to complete this assignment, which your teaching staff will explain to you.

The controlled assignment will test your understanding of the following:

- characteristics of the different life stages
- factors that have affected personal development and self-concept
- changes that have happened in a person's life
- examples of support available to clients.

In order to achieve a pass, you must show that you have knowledge of

- human development by describing the physical characteristics of different life stages (see page 132, *Human growth and development*)
- the social and economic factors that affect the development and self-concept of clients (see page 146, *Social and economic factors affecting development*, and page 155, *Self-concept*)
- relevant support available to an individual through expected life stages (see page 162, *Life changes and types of support available to those experiencing major change*).

If you are keen to gain a merit or distinction, your work will need to be more complex. Your teacher or lecturer will tell you how to achieve these higher grades.

Summary of evidence opportunities

3.1 Human growth and development

Activity A (page 138)

Case studies 1.1, 1.2, 1.3 (pages 143-144)

3.2 Social and economic factors affecting development

Activity A (page 150)

Case studies 2.1, 2.2, 2.3 (pages 152-153)

3.3 Self-concept

Activities A (page 155), B (page 157), C (page 158), D (page 159)

Case study 3.1 (page 160)

3.4 Life changes and types of support available to those experiencing major change

Activities A (page 162), B (page 165)

Case study 4.1 (page 166)

unit three

Personal evidence tracking record

Remember that you can use portfolio evidence more than once, to show understanding of other units.

3.1 Human growth and development	Description of evidence	Portfolio reference number
Infancy		
Early childhood		
Puberty and adolescence		
Adulthood		
Old age		

3.2 Factors affecting development		
Social factors		
Culture		
Gender		
Access to services		
Family		
Friends		
Housing and environment		
Ethnicity		
Isolation		
Discrimination		
Stereotyping		
Economic factors		
Income		
Effect of above factors on:		
Health		
Employment prospects		
Level of education		
Self-esteem		

3.3 Self-concept	Description of evidence	Portfolio reference number
Age		
Appearance		
Culture		
Developmental maturity		
Environment		
Education		
Gender		
Relationships		

3.4 Life changes and types of support available to those experiencing major change		
Relationship changes		
Physical changes		
Changes in location		
Linking support to individual needs		

unit three

Answers

Answers to Multiple Choice Questions, Unit One

Page 22: 1.1b 1.2a 1.3a 1.4d
Page 36: 2.1b 2.2c 2.3a 2.4d 2.5a 2.6d
Page 54: 3.1b 3.2d 3.3b 3.4c 3.5a 3.6c
Page 79: 4.1c 4.2b 4.3a 4.4d 4.5a 4.6d
        4.7c 4.8a. 4.9d 4.10d

Answers to Multiple Choice Questions, Unit Two

Page 92: 1.1b 1.2a 1.3c 1.4a
Page 110: 2.1a 2.2d 2.3c 2.4 FFTTF 2.5d 2.6c
        2.7b 2.8c
Page 125: 3.1c 3.2b 3.3a 3.4c 3.5d 3.6b 3.7b
        3.8a

Answers to Multiple Choice Questions, Unit Three

Page 145: 1.1c 1.2c 1.3a 1.4c 1.5c 1.6c
Page 154: 2.1d 2.2a 2.3c 2.4a
Page 161: 3.1d 3.2a 3.3c 3.4d
Page 167: 4.1b 4.2c 4.3d 4.4a

Answers to Crossword, page 111

Across: **1** cream cakes, **7** price, **8** salt, **11** sugar, **14** Leo, **15** tobacco, **18** can, **19** table, **20** protein, **22** Jewish, **24** mop, **27** nibble, **30** apples, **33** weans, **35** VAT, **36** red, **37** beef, **38** gnash, **40** stir, **41** vegan, **42** so, **45** vegetarians, **46** oils, **48** amiss, **51** fa, **52** ten, **54** minerals, **55** en, **56** at, **57** sugar and starch, **58** pans

Down: **2** E numbers, **3** meat, **4** kebab, **5** spice, **6** calcium, **9** lean, **10** ton, **12** rots, **13** hot pot, **16** bah, **17** clot, **21** roughage, **23** ironed, **25** pectin, **26** carbohydrates, **28** is, **29** beans, **31** press, **32** left-overs, **34** sheep, **35** vitamins, **39** hygiene, **43** lentil, **44** fare, **47** fasts, **49** menu, **50** in, **51** flan, **53** fat

Index

As the GNVQ standards are closely followed in the text, words included in them can also be found through the Contents page and the lists of 'What you need to know' at the beginning of each unit chapter.